FAST FACTS

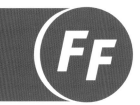

Contraception

Second edition

All You Need to
Keep up to
Speed

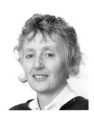

Anna Glasier MBChB BSc MD FRCOG MFFP

Director, Family Planning and Well Woman Services
NHS Lothian and University of Edinburgh
Edinburgh, UK

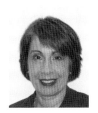

Beverly Winikoff MD MPH

President
Gynuity Health Projects
New York, USA

Declaration of Independence

This book is as balanced and as practical as we can make it. Ideas for
improvement are always welcome: feedback@fastfacts.com

D1568773

HEALTH PRESS
Oxford

Fast Facts – Contraception
First published 2000
Second edition June 2005

Text © 2005 Anna Glasier, Beverly Winikoff
© 2005 in this edition Health Press Limited
Health Press Limited, Elizabeth House, Queen Street, Abingdon,
Oxford OX14 3LN, UK
Tel: +44 (0)1235 523233
Fax: +44 (0)1235 523238

Book orders can be placed by telephone or via the website.
For regional distributors or to order via the website, please go to:
www.fastfacts.com
For telephone orders, please call 01752 202301 (UK) or
800 538 1287 (North America, toll free).

Fast Facts is a trademark of Health Press Limited.

Parts of this book, including Figures 3.1, 3.2, 8.1, 9.1 and 9.2, were adapted from
Beverly Winikoff and Suzanne Wymelenberg, *The Whole Truth about Contraception:
A Guide to Safe and Effective Choices*. Washington DC: Joseph Henry Press, 1997.

A CIP catalogue record for this title is available from the British Library.

ISBN 1-903734-46-0

Glasier A (Anna)
Fast Facts – Contraception/
Anna Glasier, Beverly Winikoff

Medical illustrations by Dee McLean, London, UK.
Typesetting and page layout by Zed, Oxford, UK.
Printed by Fine Print (Services) Ltd, Oxford, UK.

Printed with vegetable inks on fully biodegradable and
recyclable paper manufactured from sustainable forests.

444   001
Low emissions
during production

Low
chlorine

Sustainable
forests

Glossary of abbreviations

BBT: basal body temperature

CDC: Centers for Disease Control (USA)

COC: combined oral contraceptive

DMPA: depot medroxyprogesterone acetate

DVT: deep-vein thrombosis

FSH: follicle-stimulating hormone

GnRH: gonadotropin-releasing hormone

HIV: human immunodeficiency virus

HPV: human papilloma virus

IUD: intrauterine device

LAM: lactational amenorrhea method

LH: luteinizing hormone

LNG-IUS: levonorgestrel–intrauterine system

MI: myocardial infarction

PFI: pill-free interval

PMS: premenstrual syndrome

STI: sexually transmitted infection

VTE: venous thromboembolism

WHO: World Health Organization

Introduction

Most people will need to use contraception at some time in their lives. The worldwide tendency for women to delay the start of childbearing and to bear fewer children means that an increasing number will require contraception for 25 years or longer. Several contraceptive methods that are relatively cheap and easy to use are widely available, but none is perfect. Some methods are better suited to certain stages of the reproductive years and some, of course, are permanent. Even where contraception is easily accessible, unplanned pregnancies are common, most due either to failure to use a method at all or to failure to use a method correctly.

Despite the dwindling number of pharmaceutical companies involved in contraceptive development, the early 21st century has seen an increase in the number of methods available, particularly in the USA, with the arrival of new delivery systems for combined hormonal contraception, including vaginal rings, transdermal patches and the combined injectable contraceptive. An increase is also noticeable in the acceptability of long-acting methods of contraception, which rely little, if at all, on compliance for their efficacy. There is increasing evidence that long-acting methods are associated with fewer unintended pregnancies. In the USA, the depot medroxyprogesterone acetate injection (DMPA, Depo-Provera) appears to be becoming much more popular among teenagers, while among older women in the UK and continental Europe, use of the levonorgestrel-releasing intrauterine system (LNG-IUS, Mirena) is rising. An increasing awareness among users of the non-contraceptive benefits of existing methods is also apparent, especially in Europe where methods associated with amenorrhea, like the LNG-IUS, are gaining popularity.

Service providers are nowadays tending to think in terms of the wider remit of reproductive health rather than just traditional 'family planning'. Thus, the provision of contraception is enhanced by an awareness of sexual health and more attention to the prevention of sexually transmitted infections.

Although the general public appears to be reasonably knowledgeable about contraception, most people rely on well-informed professionals to help them choose an appropriate method. This book aims to provide healthcare professionals with an overview of currently available methods – how they work, their effectiveness and their side effects – and to give a description of the methods likely to become available in the relatively near future, to allow healthcare providers to anticipate new developments that may be of interest to their clients. As for the more distant future, a recently published report from the Institute of Medicine of the National Academies in the USA discusses possibilities for methods of contraception that may be developed.

Key references

Nass SJ, Strauss JF. *New Frontiers in Contraceptive Research. A blueprint for action.* Washington DC: Institute of Medicine/National Academies Press, 2001.

Stevens-Simons C, Kelly L, Kulick R. A village would be nice but ... it takes a long-acting contraceptive to prevent repeat adolescent pregnancies. *Am J Prev Med* 2001; 21:60–5.

Despite a broad choice of contraceptive methods that are not very complicated to use, unintended pregnancy is common. In the UK and USA, it is generally accepted that around 50% of women who have an unwanted pregnancy conceive while using no method of contraception. Of the 50% who conceive despite using contraception, many have not used their contraceptive method appropriately. While it is true that women take most of the responsibility for contraception, the needs and wishes of both partners must be considered if contraception is to be used effectively.

When giving advice about contraception, it is important to remember that it is a personal issue, and that contraceptive requirements will vary with different stages of a person's life. What is appropriate for a teenager may not be ideal for a perimenopausal woman. Special circumstances may make a particular method unsuitable; for example, the combined oral contraceptive pill is not recommended during lactation. Prevalence of use of the common methods of contraception in the UK and USA is shown in Figure 1.1.

When discussing contraceptive methods, three major topics should be addressed:
- safety
- efficacy/effectiveness
- acceptability.

Safety

It should never be forgotten that the object of the exercise is to avoid pregnancy. Pregnancy itself also carries risk (e.g. venous thromboembolism (VTE), pre-eclampsia and hemorrhage), and the risk is often greater than that associated with contraception. Unintended pregnancy, whether continued or not, also carries profound emotional, social and economic consequences.

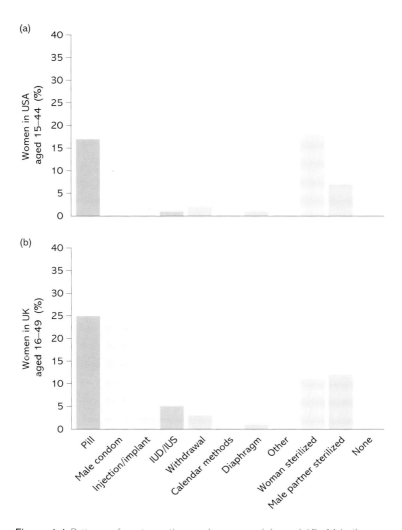

Figure 1.1 Patterns of contraceptive use by women (a) aged 15–44 in the USA (1995) and (b) aged 16–49 in the UK (2003). 'None' includes those women who are not in a heterosexual relationship, have been sterilized for non-contraceptive reasons, are trying to conceive, are pregnant or, for whatever reason (despite not wanting a baby and being at risk of conception), do not use a contraceptive. 'Other' includes the female condom, gels and foams, and emergency contraception. IUD/IUS, intrauterine device/system. USA data are from the National Survey of Family Growth (US DHHS 1997); UK data are from the Office for National Statistics Omnibus Survey (Dawe and Rainford 2004).

All methods of contraception are associated with side effects, some of which are simply a nuisance while others, albeit extremely rare, may be life-threatening. Some women may choose a less effective but safer method, while others may be prepared to accept higher risks in return for greater efficacy. The importance of individual choice should always be emphasized.

It is not easy to understand the concepts of absolute and relative risk. Many women are concerned about the risks of the combined pill and yet take much greater risks in the course of their lives (Figure 1.2). A 24% increase in the risk of breast cancer (relative

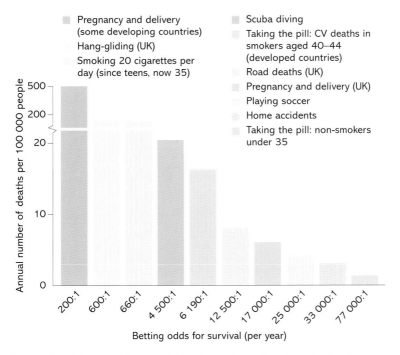

Figure 1.2 Risks associated with taking the contraceptive pill and with other activities. The risk of pill-taking for non-smokers is related to circulatory disease. With regard to cancers, the benefits of pill-taking are believed to outweigh any possible adverse effects. The risks associated with pregnancy and delivery are much higher in all countries than the risk of pill-taking for non-smokers who are under 35 years of age. CV, cardiovascular. Adapted with permission from Guillebaud J. The Pill. 5th edn. Oxford: Oxford University Press, 1997.

risk 1.24) sounds a lot. However, if the absolute risk for a woman of 20 years of age is less than 1 in 10 000 over 5 years, an increase of 24% to 1.24 in 10 000 is a level of risk that most women would accept. People's concerns about risks and side effects may sometimes seem irrational or illogical to professionals who give advice about contraception, but these concerns should be taken seriously, as they almost always affect correct use. If a woman's fears cannot be allayed, an alternative method should be discussed.

Contraindications. The World Health Organization (WHO) has published criteria for assessing an individual's medical eligibility for contraceptive use. The intention is to set international norms for providing contraception to women and men who have one or more of a range of conditions that may contraindicate one or more contraceptive methods.

Using the now-standard approach to evidence-based systematic reviews, the document (which was reviewed and updated in 2004) classifies conditions into one of four categories. Category 1 contains conditions for which there is no restriction for the use of the method, while category 4 consists of conditions which represent an unacceptable health risk if the contraceptive method is used. Classification of a method/condition as category 2 indicates that the method may generally be used but that more careful follow-up is required. Provision of a method to an individual with a category 3 condition requires careful clinical judgment and access to clinical services, since use of that method is not recommended unless there is no acceptable alternative.

The classification of headaches in relation to the use of the combined oral contraceptive pill (Table 1.1) is an example of the medical eligibility criteria tables. The document is not meant to provide rigid guidelines, but rather gives recommendations to be adapted in the light of national health policies, need and resources. The document is available on the web (www.who.int/reproductive-health/publications/MEC_3/mec.pdf), and a system is in place to incorporate new evidence into the guidelines as it becomes available.

TABLE 1.1

Extract from the World Health Organization (WHO) *Medical Eligibility Criteria for Contraceptive Use* 2004

Use of the low-dose combined oral contraceptive pill (≤ 35 µg ethinyl estradiol) by women with neurological conditions

Headaches	Initiation	Continuation	Comments, new evidence
Non-migrainous (mild or severe)	1	2	**Comments:** Classification depends on accurate diagnosis of those severe headaches that are migrainous and those that are not. Any new headaches or marked changes in headaches should be evaluated. Classification is for women without any other risk factors for stroke. Risk of stroke increases with age, hypertension and smoking.
Migraine			
(i) without aura			
Age < 35	2	3	
Age ≥ 35	3	4	**Evidence:** Among women with migraine, women who also had aura had a higher risk of stroke than those without aura. In addition, among women with migraine, those who used combined oral contraceptives had a two- to fourfold increased risk of stroke compared with women who did not use combined oral contraceptives.
(ii) with aura			
(at any age)	4	4	

1, no restriction; 2, advantages outweigh risks; 3, caution, risks usually outweigh advantages; 4, contraindication, unacceptable health risk.
Reproduced with permission from WHO. *Medical Eligibility Criteria for Contraceptive Use*. 3rd edn. Geneva: Reproductive Health and Research, World Health Organization, 2004. Also available on the web at www.who.int/reproductive-health/publications/MEC_3/mec.pdf.

Efficacy and effectiveness

'Efficacy' means the inherent ability of the method to prevent pregnancy; 'effectiveness' refers to typical use, when factors such as compliance affect the efficacy. Failure rates are usually given as the percentage of women who experience an unintended pregnancy in the first year of perfect use (i.e. the method is used perfectly but conception occurs) and of typical use.

No method of contraception is 100% effective. People get better at using a method with time but, of course, the cumulative probability of becoming pregnant increases with time. The cumulative pregnancy rate (the probability of getting pregnant over a given period of contraceptive use) is particularly relevant when considering the efficacy of a long-acting contraceptive, such as the intrauterine device (IUD). Table 1.2 summarizes the effectiveness of currently available contraceptive methods.

In 2002 WHO produced a second evidence-based document providing guidance on the safe and effective use of contraception, which was revised and extended in 2004 (http://www.who.int/ reproductive-health/publications/rhr_02_7/spr.pdf). Like the WHO *Medical Eligibility Criteria for Contraceptive Use*, these *Selected Practice Recommendations for Contraceptive Use* (SPR) are meant to be adapted to suit the needs and resources of different countries. The document covers 23 specific questions derived from controversies or inconsistencies in existing guidance. It gives advice on the time in the menstrual cycle when contraceptive methods can be started without significant risk of pregnancy; what to do about missed pills or late injections; which tests or examinations are routinely required before a method can be provided; and how often to follow up users. The document is aimed primarily at developing countries, where resources are often limited and where the benefits of relaxing some of the prescribing advice to allow widespread access to contraception for many thousands of couples outweighs the risks of occasional pregnancy and rare complications. In settings where the prevalence of contraception is high (and litigation common), as in many developed countries, the recommendations will seem to some to be too lax. With this in mind, the Faculty of

TABLE 1.2

Effectiveness of contraceptive methods: percentage of women experiencing an unintended pregnancy during the first year of use and percentage continuing use at the end of the first year (USA)

Method	% pregnant		% continuing
	Typical use	Perfect use	
No method	85	85	
Spermicides	29	18	42
Withdrawal	27	4	43
Periodic abstinence	25		51
Calendar		9	
Ovulation method		3	
Symptothermal		2	
Postovulation		1	
Cap, parous women	32	26	46
nulliparous women	16	9	57
Sponge, parous women	32	20	46
nulliparous women	16	9	57
Diaphragm	16	6	57
Condom, female (Reality)	21	5	49
male	15	2	53
Combined pill and minipill*	8	0.3	68
Combined hormonal patch (Evra)	8	0.3	68
Combined hormonal ring (NuvaRing)	8	0.3	68
DMPA (Depo-Provera)	3	0.3	56
Combined injectable (Lunelle)	3	0.05	56
IUD, copper T (ParaGard)	0.8	0.6	78
LNG-IUS (Mirena)	0.1	0.1	81
LNG implant (Norplant, Norplant-2)	0.05	0.05	84
Female sterilization	0.5	0.5	100
Male sterilization	0.15	0.10	100

Emergency contraceptive pills taken within 72 hours of unprotected intercourse reduce the risk of pregnancy by at least 75%

Lactational amenorrhea is a highly effective, *temporary* contraceptive method

*Combined pills have a lower failure rate than the progestogen-only minipill (page 48). Adapted with permission from Trussell J. Contraceptive efficacy. In Hatcher RA et al. 2004.

Family Planning and Reproductive Healthcare of the Royal
College of Obstetricians and Gynaecologists in the UK held a
consensus meeting of experts designed to adapt or adopt the
recommendations for use in the UK; the conclusions are available
at www.ffprhc.org.uk/Key%20Points%20final1.pdf.

Acceptability

Although the acceptability of a method is inextricably linked to
both its efficacy and safety, many other factors determine whether
an individual person finds a particular method acceptable or not.
There is always a balance to be found between the advantages of
a particular method and the disadvantages. Minor side effects and
inconvenience are particularly important in this respect. Many
women tolerate irregular bleeding with the subdermal levonorgestrel
implant (Norplant) because protection lasts for 5 years, it is
extremely effective and the user does not have to remember to
do anything. In contrast, the same women may not accept the
same bleeding pattern with the progestogen-only pill because of its
lower efficacy and the need to remember to take a pill every day.

The consultation

Most women – and it is usually the woman who attends a
contraceptive consultation – are relatively well informed about
contraception, although many may not understand the mode of
action of particular contraceptive methods or have a clear idea
of efficacy. The provision of contraception is often straightforward,
and most people seeking advice are fit and well. It is easy to
overmedicalize contraception, particularly when the consultation
is used as an opportunity for health screening, such as
performing cervical (Pap) smears. Nonetheless, some methods of
contraception have potentially dangerous (although fortunately
rare) consequences, and care should be taken to note any factors in
the personal or family history that may increase these risks. Use
of the WHO *Medical Eligibility Criteria* may be helpful in this
context. Other health benefits – for example, the beneficial effect of
the combined pill for dysmenorrhea and premenstrual syndrome

(PMS) – should be stressed, and the approach should be a holistic one. Wherever appropriate, discussions about a method should be broadened to include safe sex and other reproductive health issues. It is important to assess an individual's risks of sexually transmitted infection (STI) when helping him or her choose an appropriate method of contraception. For example, an IUD is not the most appropriate method for a woman with multiple partners.

Ultimately, the aim should be to allow the contraceptive user to make an informed choice of a method with which she or he feels confident and safe, and that she or he knows how to use correctly.

Key points – consultation

- Most people use contraception at some stage in their lives.
- Contraceptive needs – and therefore the suitability of the available methods – change with different stages of each person's reproductive life.
- Contraception is essentially safe; it is the *perceived* risk that often deters people from using a method.
- Methods that place demands on compliance for effectiveness have higher failure rates.
- Long-acting methods, because they make few or no demands on the user, have lower failure rates.
- The World Health Organization publishes a set of regularly updated evidence-based guidelines for safe and effective contraceptive use.

Key references

Dawe F, Rainford L. *Contraception and Sexual Health 2003*. London. Office for National Statistics, 2004.

Glasier A, Brechin S, Raine R, Penney G. A consensus process to adapt the WHO Selected Practice Recommendations for UK use. *Contraception* 2003;68:327–33.

Glasier A, Gebbie A. *Handbook of Family Planning and Reproductive Health Care*. 4th edn. Edinburgh: Churchill Livingstone, 2000.

Hatcher RA, Trussell J, Stewart F et al. *Contraceptive Technology*, 18th edn. New York: Ardent Media, 2004.

Larsson G, Blohm F, Sundell G et al. A longitudinal study of birth control and pregnancy outcome among women in a Swedish population. *Contraception* 1997;56:9–16.

Piccinino LJ, Mosher WD. Trend in contraceptive use in the United States 1982–1995. *Fam Plann Perspect* 1998;30:4–10,46.

Rosenberg A, Waugh MS. Causes and consequences of oral contraceptive non-compliance. *Am J Obstet Gynecol* 1999;180:276–9.

Scott A, Glasier A. Are routine breast and pelvic examinations necessary for women starting combined oral contraception? *Hum Reprod Update* 2004;10:449–52.

US Department of Health and Human Services. *Fertility, Family Planning and Women's Health: New Data from the 1995 National Survey of Family Growth*. NCHS Series 23, No. 19. Washington: US Department of Health and Human Services, Centers for Disease Control and Prevention, National Center for Health Statistics, 1997.

WHO. *Medical Eligibility Criteria for Contraceptive Use*. 3rd edn. Geneva: Reproductive Health and Research, World Health Organization, 2004. www.who.int/reproductive-health/publications/MEC_3/mec.pdf

WHO. *Selected Practice Recommendations*. Geneva: Reproductive Health and Research, World Health Organization, 2004. Also available on the web at www.who.int/reproductive-health/publications/rhr_02_7/spr.pdf

Wilcox AJ, Weinberg CR, Baird DD. Timing of sexual intercourse in relation to ovulation. Effects on the probability of conception, survival of the pregnancy and sex of the baby. *N Engl J Med* 1995;333:1517–21.

Winikoff B, Wymelenberg S. *The Whole Truth About Contraception. A Guide to Safe and Effective Choices*. Washington: Joseph Henry, 1997.

Cycle-based fertility awareness methods

These methods are based on the knowledge that the only time when fertilization is likely is during the 8–10 days in the middle of a typical menstrual cycle. Although menstrual cycles vary in length, the 'fertile phase' is almost always the same length. Successful use of cycle-based birth control depends on learning which cycle days are fertile and either refraining from penetrative intercourse or using another form of contraception on these days. An abstinence approach can mean avoiding penetrative sex for one-third to one-half of the month. Traditional fertility-observation methods have no negative physical side effects, and the costs are low to the user. The disadvantage is that, to be successful, these methods require real commitment and diligent practice.

Physiological basis. Early in the cycle, the pituitary releases follicle-stimulating hormone (FSH), which stimulates a number of follicles in the ovary to grow and secrete estrogen. This causes the cervix to produce more mucus. The cervical os widens as the mucus becomes abundant, watery and 'stretchy'. The increased level of estrogen also stimulates the pituitary to secrete luteinizing hormone (LH). The resulting surge of LH triggers the release of a mature ovum from its follicle, which then begins to produce progesterone. Stimulation by this hormone causes changes in both the quality and the quantity of cervical mucus, and increases the basal body temperature (BBT). Temperature remains measurably elevated until progesterone level declines. When the progesterone concentration falls, the endometrium begins to be sloughed off, menstruation occurs and the cycle begins again (see Figure 5.2, page 47). Ovulation occurs approximately 14 days before the onset of menstruation, regardless of the total length of a woman's menstrual cycle.

Ova are viable for only 12–24 hours, but sperm can survive in the reproductive tract for as long as 7 days. Ovulation predictor kits, available in pharmacies and drug stores, can detect ovulation 24–48 hours beforehand – not soon enough to alert a couple to avoid intercourse, considering the survival ability of sperm. In the UK, a computerized monitor (Persona) is available that takes readings of urinary hormone levels and predicts safe (green light) and unsafe (red light) days. The monitor reads red on 6–10 days a month, indicating the need for a barrier method or abstinence to avoid pregnancy.

Efficacy. It is difficult to establish an accurate failure rate for cycle-based methods. They work better for highly motivated, older couples who have used them for a while. Among perfect users, first-year failure rates vary from 1 to 9%. Among typical users, however, 20–25% become pregnant during the first year.

Calendar/rhythm method. A calendar of at least eight menstrual cycles is made. To calculate fertile days, subtract 18 from the length of the shortest cycle and 11 from the length of the longest cycle. These two numbers represent the beginning and the end of the fertile days.

Temperature method. BBT, or resting temperature, is charted for 3 or 4 months to establish fertility patterns. After ovulation, the BBT usually rises by between 0.22 and 0.44°C (0.4 and 0.8°F) and remains at that level until just before menstruation begins. A woman can consider herself to be safely not fertile after 3 days of raised temperature. BBT is taken in the morning before rising and prior to eating or drinking. It can be measured orally, rectally or vaginally, but the same method should be used every time. Because the temperature rise is triggered by progesterone after ovulation, this method cannot be used to warn of ovulation. Illness, alcohol consumption and a later rising time can raise the BBT.

Cervical mucus method. Changes in mucus can signal the onset of the fertile period. The cervical glands secrete very little mucus immediately following menstruation. After a few 'dry' days, the mucus remains scant, but becomes sticky and appears somewhat white, yellow or cloudy. When this type of mucus is present, unprotected intercourse is no longer safe.

A few days before ovulation, the mucus becomes much more abundant, clear, slippery and very 'stretchy'. The last day on which this type of mucus occurs is the day of peak fertility. Peak fertility has only definitely passed when the mucus returns to being sticky and scant (3–4 days after the peak fertility day). Women are not fertile from this time until after menstruation and when the fertile phase of the next cycle begins. Vaginal infections, douching or any use of lubricant or spermicidal jelly will make it difficult to interpret mucus changes.

Symptothermal method. This combines checking cervical mucus, recording BBT and watching for the other signs of ovulation. For example, during the infertile phase, the cervix is lower in the vagina, easier to reach and firm to the touch. As ovulation approaches, the cervix becomes higher, broader and softer. After ovulation, the cervix is again low in the vagina and feels firm and closed. The infertile period begins:

- after 3 days of increased BBT
- after 3 days of a closed, firm, low cervix
- 4 days after the peak fertility day.

This combined approach is particularly useful for women with unusually short or long cycles.

Breastfeeding

Many women, and even some doctors, are not aware that exclusive breastfeeding can be very effective in pregnancy prevention. Lactation delays the body's return to its usual cycle of ovulation (Figure 2.1), sometimes for as long as a year, depending on how often the baby is nursed. When lactational amenorrhea is deliberately used to prevent pregnancy, it is referred to as the lactational amenorrhea method (LAM). This can be continued for some months after childbirth and is a very effective method of contraception. For women who breastfeed exclusively, have no

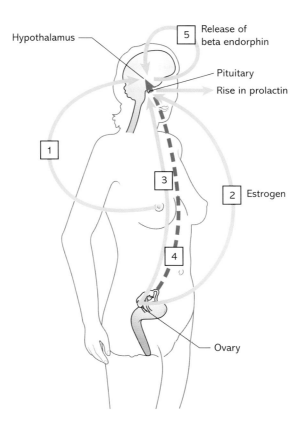

Figure 2.1 Possible mechanisms of lactational amenorrhea:
(1) nerve impulses from the nipple produce a rise in the level of prolactin produced by the pituitary, but also
(2) changed hypothalamic sensitivity to ovarian steroid feedback and
(3) altered gonadotropin secretion.
(4) Whether prolactin contributes directly to the changes in hypothalamic sensitivity or blocks gonadotropin activity at the level of the ovary is not established.
(5) Suckling may also stimulate the release of beta endorphin, which suppresses gonadotropin-releasing hormone from the hypothalamus.
Adapted with permission from *Contraception During Breastfeeding: A Clinician's Sourcebook.* 2nd edn. New York: Population Council, 1997.

signs of menstruation and have not passed the 6-month postpartum mark, the risk of pregnancy while relying on LAM is less than 2% (Figure 2.2). Lactational amenorrhea can be maintained by ensuring that the intervals between nursing are not longer than 4 hours and that almost all of the baby's nutrition comes from breast milk.

It is a good idea for women to use a contraceptive as soon as they start giving supplemental foods, because there is a risk that a fertile first ovulation will occur before any sign of menstruation. Many contraceptive methods can be used safely during breastfeeding. Condoms and spermicides pose no risk to either mother or child; furthermore, condoms offer protection against infection. It is necessary to wait until the uterus and cervix have returned to normal size and position before fitting a diaphragm or cervical cap. Intrauterine devices are suitable for breastfeeding women; the risk of expulsion is reduced if the device is inserted after the uterus has returned to its normal size, about 6 weeks after birth. Less discomfort seems to occur when insertion takes place while the woman is still breastfeeding.

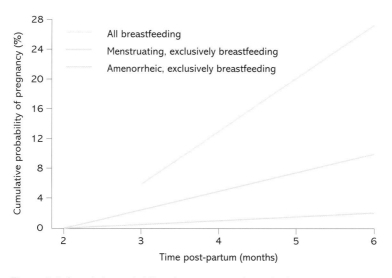

Figure 2.2 Cumulative probability of pregnancy in breastfeeding women. Reproduced with permission from *Contraception During Breastfeeding: A Clinician's Sourcebook.* 2nd edn. New York: Population Council, 1997.

Combined oral contraceptives are not recommended for breastfeeding women. The estrogen in the combined pill decreases milk supply, which may lead to earlier use of supplemental feeding and to early weaning. Progestogen-only methods – depot medroxyprogesterone acetate, progestogen-only pills, progestogen-releasing IUDs and the subdermal levonorgestrel implant – are safe for the baby and do not negatively affect milk production or infant growth. However, the hormones are excreted in breast milk.

Tubal occlusion and vasectomy are effective methods of contraception while a woman is breastfeeding. Fertility awareness methods are not ideal during nursing, because the patterns of cervical mucus and BBT are not typical during this time and may be hard to discern.

Key points – biologically based methods

- A woman's monthly hormonal cycle produces observable clues to her fertility.
- Couples can use knowledge of female physiology to avoid pregnancy.
- Biologically based methods are heavily dependent on individual behavior for effectiveness.
- Methods based on periodic abstinence tend to have high failure rates when used typically.
- Exclusive breastfeeding is an effective method of contraception for up to 6 months after parturition.
- Women can combine breastfeeding with any of a number of other methods for enhanced effectiveness, especially after 6 months postpartum or return of menses.

Key references

Arevalo M, Jennings V, Sinai I. Application of simple fertility awareness-based methods of family planning to breastfeeding women. *Fertil Steril* 2003;80:1241–8.

Billings E, Westmore A. *The Billings Method*. New York: Random House, 1980.

Breastfeeding and contraception. *Outlook* 1990;8:2–10.

Diaz S, Seron-Ferre M, Croxatto HB, Veldhuis J. Neuroendocrine mechanisms of lactational infertility in women. *Biol Res* 1995;28:155–63.

Freundl G, Godehardt E, Kern PA et al. Estimated maximum failure rates of cycle monitors using daily conception probabilities in the menstrual cycle. *Hum Reprod* 2003;18:2628–33.

Hight-Laukaran V, Labbok MH, Peterson AE et al. Multicenter study of the Lactational Amenorrhea Method (LAM): II. Acceptability, utility and policy implications. *Contraception* 1997;55:337–46.

Kennedy KI, Gross BA, Van Look PFA. Lactational amenorrhea method for family planning. *Int J Gynecol Obstet* 1996;54:55–7.

Labbok MH, Hight-Laukaran V, Peterson AE et al. Multicenter study of the Lactational Amenorrhea Method (LAM): I. Efficacy, duration and implications for clinical application. *Contraception* 1997;55: 327–36.

McNeilly AS. Lactational control of reproduction. *Reprod Fertil Dev* 2001;13:583–90.

Rous JJ. Is breast-feeding a substitute for contraception in family planning? *Demography* 2001;38:497–512.

Trussell J, Grummer-Strawn L. Contraceptive failure of the ovulation method of periodic abstinence. *Fam Plann Perspect* 1990;22:65–75.

Van Look PFA. Lactational amenorrhoea method for family planning. *BMJ* 1996; 313:893–4.

Winikoff B, Semeraro P, Zimmerman M, Stein K. *Contraception During Breast-feeding: A Clinician's Sourcebook*. New York: Population Council, 1997.

Barrier methods create a physical barrier (condoms, diaphragm, cervical cap) or chemical barrier (spermicide) that blocks sperm from fertilizing an ovum. They are the only contraceptives shown to prevent STIs; only condoms have been shown to prevent human immunodeficiency virus (HIV) infection. The male condom is the most commonly used barrier method.

Condoms and spermicides are available without a prescription, whereas most diaphragms and cervical caps require prescription from a health professional.

Male condoms

Condoms may be made of latex, polyurethane or, in the USA, treated animal tissue. They do not require a prescription and can be used with a spermicide. Uncircumcised men need to pull the foreskin back before putting on the condom. Although some men complain that wearing a condom diminishes pleasure, others find that a small decrease in stimulation allows them to prolong sexual play.

Condoms have a failure rate of 3–12%; those that have been stored for a long period are more likely to break. In the UK, condoms that display the British kitemark on the packaging meet guaranteed standards.

Emergency contraception is available to prevent pregnancy after condom breakage and slippage (see Chapter 7).

Latex condoms are the most widely available and least expensive. These condoms have been shown to provide very good protection from STIs, including HIV infection. Allergy to latex products or the spermicide that coats some condoms is fairly common, however.

If additional lubrication is desired, it is important to use only water or a water-based lubricant. Oils and grease react with the latex and weaken it.

Polyurethane condoms have been approved for sale in the USA and the UK. Polyurethane transfers body heat readily, so there is more sensation during sex. These condoms are much more expensive than latex ones but are preferable if either partner has a latex allergy.

'Skin' condoms are made from treated lamb membranes. They are thinner and stronger than latex, and some men believe they permit more sensation. However, skin condoms do not protect against disease, as the membrane's pores, though too small for sperm to pass through, are large enough to allow the passage of microorganisms.

Spermicide

Spermicide is available as foam, gel or cream, with applicators, and as dissolvable suppositories or squares of film (Table 3.1). Some spermicidal products are made to be used with a diaphragm or cervical cap. The active ingredient in all these formulations is nonoxynol-9, which works by damaging the surface membrane of the sperm cell.

Spermicidal products are available over the counter. They are inserted before intercourse and can seldom be distinguished from the natural lubrication of the vagina. Some products require at least a 15-minute wait so they can melt. Most are effective for only 1 hour; for a second act of intercourse after more than 1 hour, another application is needed. For typical users, spermicide used alone (without a condom) has a first-year failure rate from 6 to 21%.

Spermicide provides some protection against *Chlamydia* and gonorrhea, and possibly also against cervical cancer and hepatitis B virus infection. Nonoxynol-9 kills HIV and herpes viruses in vitro, but its in-vivo efficacy has not been demonstrated.

The most common health problem associated with spermicide is irritation of the penis or vagina. Irritation caused by nonoxynol-9 may be associated with increased risk of HIV infection among frequent (multiple times per day) users of spermicidal products. For this reason, the WHO and the Centers for Disease Control (CDC,

TABLE 3.1

Spermicidal products available in the UK and USA*

Jellies, gels and creams

- Conceptrol Gel Disposables (prefilled applicators) (USA)
- Duragel (UK)
- Koromex Jelly (USA)
- Koromex Crystal Clear Gel[†] (USA)
- Gynol II Original Formula jelly[†] – no applicator included (USA and UK)
- Gynol II Extra Strength (USA)
- Ortho-Creme (USA and UK)

Foams

- Delfen contraceptive foam (USA and UK)
- Koromex Foam (USA)

Vaginal suppositories

- Koromex Vaginal Inserts[‡] (USA)
- Conceptrol Inserts[‡] (USA)
- Semicid[‡] (USA)
- Encare[‡] (USA)
- Orthoforms (UK)

Contraceptive film

- Vaginal Contraceptive Film (VCF)[†] (USA)

Bioadhesive gel

- Advantage 24 – prefilled applicators (USA)

*The active ingredient in all these products is nonoxynol-9.
[†]To be used only in conjunction with a diaphragm or condom.
[‡]Requires 10–15 minutes to melt before it becomes effective.

USA) have recommended that such products not be used for contraception by women at high risk of HIV infection, especially if the products will be used frequently. In addition, use of spermicidal products for lubrication during anal sex is strongly discouraged. Since addition of nonoxynol-9 to condoms does not increase their effectiveness for contraception or disease prevention, it is recommended that such condoms no longer be promoted or sold.

Early reports of an association between the use of spermicide after conception and the risk of spontaneous abortion or of bearing a child with birth defects were not substantiated in later studies.

Diaphragm

The diaphragm is a round, shallow rubber cap with a flexible spring rim. It is used with a spermicide and fits snugly across the upper vagina, covering the cervix. Diaphragms are available in diameters from 50 to 95 mm. The size needed is related to body size, weight and parity. A trained healthcare professional carries out the fitting, using rings or sample diaphragms. The ideal device is the largest size that is snug without discomfort, touching the walls of the vagina with just enough room to insert a fingertip beneath the pubic bone. The fitting procedure includes a lesson on how to insert and remove the diaphragm. The diaphragm is inserted, with spermicide in the cup, before intercourse, and it should remain in place for 6 hours afterwards. Diaphragms can be used during menstruation.

A diaphragm offers protection against pregnancy, bacterial STIs, cervical cancer and pelvic inflammatory disease. Protection against HIV and other viruses has not yet been demonstrated; research under way on these issues should provide more definitive information within the next few years. Some women who wear diaphragms experience repeated urinary tract infections, possibly owing to the pressure of the rim on the urethra and bladder. Diaphragm users or their partners may be allergic to the latex or spermicide.

Failure rates vary from 5 to 21% during the first year. Diaphragms should be examined every few weeks for holes, and the fit should be checked after:

- loss or gain of more than about 9 kg (20 pounds) in weight
- childbirth
- miscarriage

- abortion
- pelvic surgery
- recurring bladder infection.

It should also be checked if the user suspects it does not fit.

Cervical caps

The cervical cap is a small latex cup with a firm, flexible rim. It is 32–38 mm long (1.25–1.5 inches) and looks like a large rubber thimble. The cap is available in four different inside diameters and fits snugly over the cervix, held in place by suction. For a good fit, the inner diameter of the cap must be only 1–2 mm larger than the cervix (Figure 3.1), and the cap should not rest right on the os. About 20% of women cannot get a good fit. In the USA, a cervical smear is recommended before a cap is fitted and after 3 months of use.

The cap (plus spermicide) protects against some STIs. It has not been shown to protect against HIV infection. As the cervical cap is latex, it can be damaged by any oil-based substance. It may also irritate the cervix or the penis mechanically or because of latex allergy. It cannot be used during menstruation because it does not permit any flow of secretions.

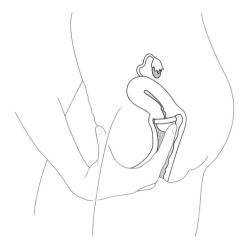

Figure 3.1 Checking placement of the cap.

The cervical cap is used with spermicide placed in its dome. It should be inserted at least 20 minutes before intercourse so that a good seal can develop. If the cap becomes displaced, women are advised to apply spermicide immediately; emergency contraception should be recommended. After intercourse, the cap is left in place for at least 6 hours. There is a theoretical risk of toxic shock syndrome if the cap is worn for more than 72 hours, although no documented cases exist.

When the cap is exposed to vaginal secretions it develops an odor, but this can be neutralized by soaking in lemon juice or vinegar solution. Caps usually need to be replaced every 12–18 months. Failure rates range from 8 to 19% during the first year of use.

Lea's shield. A variant of the cervical cap called Lea's shield was approved by the US Food and Drug Administration (FDA) in March 2002. It is also available over the counter in Canada and parts of Europe, but not in the UK. Because it comes in only one size, it does not require fitting. This silicone device is washable and reusable for about a year and has a one-way valve to allow cervical secretions to be discharged without removal of the cap. According to its manufacturers, the cap is to be used with spermicide and has a 1-year effectiveness rate of 95%. The shield should stay in place after intercourse for 6 to 8 hours, but the device should not be left in the vagina for more than 48 hours. It is recommended that a cervical smear be performed after a woman has been using Lea's shield for 6 months.

FemCap. The most recent addition to the array of cervical caps in both the USA and the UK is called the FemCap. The device consists of a dome that fits over the cervix and a flanged brim that extends down along the vagina (Figure 3.2). A strap is attached to the dome for removal. The FemCap comes in three sizes (inner rim diameter 22, 26 and 30 mm), the smallest intended for women who have never been pregnant, the medium for women who have been pregnant but have not had a vaginal delivery and the largest for

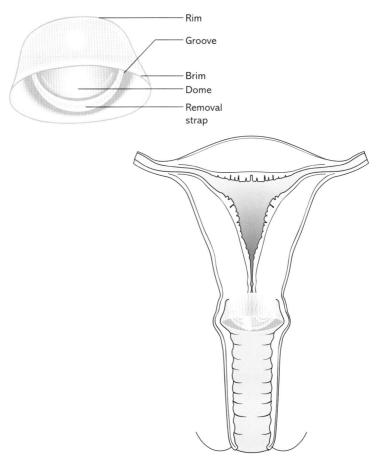

Figure 3.2 The FemCap and its position.

women who have had a vaginal delivery of a full-term baby. There is a groove between the dome and the brim to allow placement of spermicide. The FemCap is more difficult to insert and remove, and less effective than a standard diaphragm.

Female condoms

The female condom is a soft, loose-fitting polyurethane pouch, approximately 7.5 cm (3 inches) in diameter and 15 cm (6 inches) long, lubricated both inside and out (Figure 3.3). It looks like a miniature windsock and is designed to line the vagina. There is a

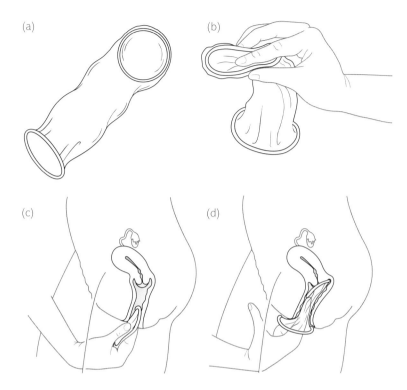

Figure 3.3 Inserting the female condom. (a) The condom unrolled. (b) The condom in the position for insertion, with the inner ring pinched. (c) The condom is inserted as shown. (d) The inner ring is placed high in the vagina, covering the cervix.

flexible ring at each end; the slightly smaller ring at the closed end is placed over the cervix. The ring at the open end remains about 2.5 cm (1 inch) outside the vagina. Like the male condom, each condom should be used once only.

As the female condom is made from polyurethane, it is less likely to tear or cause allergy than latex. It is not affected by oil-based substances and transfers body heat easily, permitting more sensation. It does not require the use of a spermicide. Viruses have not been able to penetrate the polyurethane in laboratory tests. The annual rate of pregnancy is listed as 5% for perfect users and 21% for typical users.

Currently, only one version of the female condom is available over the counter in the UK (Femidom). In the USA, female condoms (FC Female Condom and Femidom) can be bought over the internet and in retail outlets.

Contraindications

There are virtually no contraindications (category 4 listings) in the WHO *Medical Eligibility Criteria* for barrier methods. The only cautions (category 3) pertain to latex allergy for certain condoms, diaphragms and cervical caps, and for history of toxic shock syndrome for users of the diaphragm and cervical cap.

Key points – barrier methods

• Barrier methods are the only contraceptives that have been shown to protect against sexually transmitted infections.

• All barrier methods require planning and use at the time of intercourse.

• The male condom is the only reversible form of contraceptive for men.

• Spermicides should not be used for contraception by women at high risk of HIV infection or during anal sex.

• With consistent use, barrier methods provide effective contraception.

• Barrier methods present almost no health risks to users.

Key references

Alexander NJ. Barriers to sexually transmitted diseases. *Sci Am Med Sci* 1996;3:32–41.

Cates W Jr, Steiner MJ. Dual protection against unintended pregnancy and sexually transmitted infections: what is the best contraceptive approach? *Sex Transm Dis* 2002;29:168–74.

Cates W Jr. The NIH condom report: the glass is 90% full. *Fam Plann Perspect* 2001;33:231–3.

Centers for Disease Control and Prevention. *Facts About Condoms and Their Use in Preventing HIV Infection and Other STDs*. Atlanta: CDC, 1995.

Cook L, Nanda K, Grimes D. Diaphragm versus diaphragm with spermicides for contraception. *Cochrane Database Syst Rev* 2003;1:CD002031 (www.thecochranelibrary.com); The diaphragm with and without spermicide for contraception: a Cochrane review. *Hum Reprod* 2002;17:867–9.

Gallo MF, Grimes DA, Schulz KF. Nonlatex vs. latex male condoms for contraception: a systematic review of randomized controlled trials. *Contraception* 2003;68:319–26.

Gallo MF, Grimes DA, Schulz KF. Cervical cap versus diaphragm for contraception. *Cochrane Database Syst Rev* 2002;4:CD003551. (www.thecochranelibrary.com).

Gollub EL, French P, Latka M et al. Achieving safer sex with choice: studying a women's sexual risk reduction hierarchy in an STD clinic. *J Womens Health Gend Based Med* 2001;10:771–83.

Kuyoh MA, Toroitich-Ruto C, Grimes DA et al. Sponge versus diaphragm for contraception: a Cochrane review. *Contraception* 2003;67:15–18; *Cochrane Database Syst Rev* 2002;3:CD003172 (www.thecochranelibrary.com).

Mauck C, Callahan M, Weiner DH, Dominik R. The FemCap Investigators' Group. A comparative study of the safety and efficacy of FemCap, a new vaginal barrier contraceptive, and the Ortho All-Flex diaphragm. *Contraception* 1999; 60:71–80.

Ness RB, Soper DE, Holley RL et al. Hormonal and barrier contraception and risk of upper genital tract disease in the PID Evaluation and Clinical Health (PEACH) study. *Am J Obstet Gynecol* 2001;185:121–7.

Raymond EG, Chen PL, Luoto J. Spermicide Trial Group. Contraceptive effectiveness and safety of five nonoxynol-9 spermicides: a randomized trial. *Obstet Gynecol* 2004;103:430–9.

Trussell J, Strickler J, Vaughan B. Contraceptive efficacy of the diaphragm, the sponge and the cervical cap. *Fam Plann Perspect* 1993;25:100–5.

Warner DL, Hatcher RA. A meta-analysis of condom effectiveness in reducing sexually transmitted HIV. *Soc Sci Med* 1994;38:1169–70.

Wilkinson D, Tholandi M, Ramjee G, Rutherford GW. Nonoxynol-9 spermicide for prevention of vaginally acquired HIV and other sexually transmitted infections: systematic review and meta-analysis of randomised controlled trials including more than 5000 women. *Lancet Infect Dis* 2002;2:613–17.

World Health Organization. WHO/CONRAD technical consultation on nonoxynol-9, World Health Organization, Geneva, 9–10 October 2001: summary report. *Reprod Health Matters* 2002; 10:175–81.

Intrauterine devices (IUDs) have been used throughout the world since the early 1960s. Early models like the Lippes loop were made of polyurethane. The addition of copper to the device improved efficacy, allowing the development of smaller IUDs with fewer side effects, particularly menorrhagia and dysmenorrhea. Modern, second-generation copper devices have either more copper wire than their predecessors, or copper sleeves and/or a copper wire with a silver core, with the result that they last longer and are more effective. In the UK, where some 7% of couples using contraception rely on an IUD, seven different copper IUDs are currently available, varying in shape, size and the amount of copper they bear. In the USA, bad publicity damaged the reputation of the IUD during the 1980s, and nowadays fewer than 1% of American women using contraception use an IUD. Reflecting this decline in popularity, only one copper model (the ParaGard T 380A) is currently available in the USA. Copper IUDs last for approximately 10 years.

A frameless IUD is available in the UK. It comprises six copper beads threaded on to a non-biodegradable polypropylene thread; the top and bottom beads are crimped to keep all the beads in place. The upper end of the thread is knotted and embedded to a depth of 1 cm into the fundal myometrium (Figure 4.1). Efficacy appears to be equivalent to the framed copper models, but expulsion rates and removals for pain and bleeding are lower.

One hormone-releasing IUD is available. The Mirena system has a sleeve of the progestogen levonorgestrel around its stem; it releases 20 µg levonorgestrel per day and lasts for at least 5 years (Figure 4.2). Marketed as an intrauterine system (IUS) to distinguish it from non-medicated devices, Mirena has been available for contraception in the UK since the mid-1990s and for the treatment of idiopathic menorrhagia since 2001. In the USA it is not yet licensed for treating menorrhagia but has been approved for contraception since December 2000.

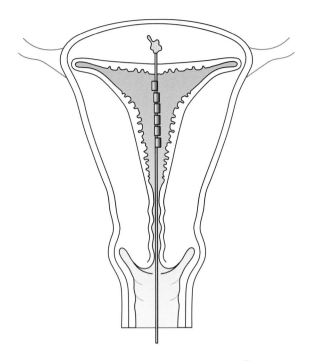

Figure 4.1 The frameless intrauterine device in position. The knot is embedded in the myometrium by means of a special insertion device.

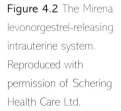

Figure 4.2 The Mirena levonorgestrel-releasing intrauterine system. Reproduced with permission of Schering Health Care Ltd.

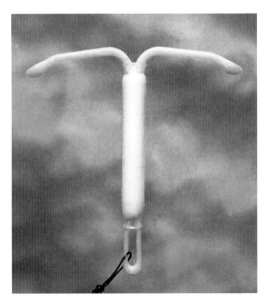

Mechanism of action

Copper intrauterine devices stimulate an inflammatory reaction in the uterus. The concentrations of macrophages, leukocytes, prostaglandins and various enzymes in both uterine and tubal fluid increase significantly. It is thought that these effects are toxic to both sperm and egg and also interfere with sperm transport. The effects on the endometrium almost certainly prevent implantation should a healthy, fertilized egg reach the uterine cavity.

Hormone-releasing systems produce endometrial atrophy and change the characteristics of cervical mucus. Ovarian activity is not inhibited, but, as with all low-dose progestogen-only methods, ovarian follicles tend to persist, and cycles tend to have inadequate or short luteal phases. The manufacturers of Mirena state that its contraceptive effect is largely the result of its effect on cervical mucus.

Efficacy

The probabilities of pregnancy during the first year of IUD use and the cumulative pregnancy rates after 7 years of use are shown in Table 4.1.

Contraindications

There are few contraindications in the WHO *Medical Eligibility Criteria* to an intrauterine device. Conditions which are classified as category 4 (contraindication; an unacceptable health risk) for both copper IUDs and the LNG-IUS (Mirena) are listed in Table 4.2.

TABLE 4.1

The efficacy of intrauterine contraceptives

	Cumulative pregnancy rate in first year (%)	Cumulative pregnancy rate at 7 years (%)
Copper IUD	0.6	1.7
Levonorgestrel IUS	0.1	1.1

TABLE 4.2

WHO *Medical Eligibility Criteria* 2004 category 4 conditions (absolute contraindications) for use of copper IUDs and the LNG-IUS

Condition	Category	
	Cu IUD	LNG-IUS
Pregnancy	4	4
Puerperal sepsis	4	4
Immediate post-septic abortion	4	4
Anatomic abnormalities that distort the uterine cavity	4	4
Fibroids that distort the uterine cavity	4	4
Unexplained vaginal bleeding before evaluation	I 4, C 2	I 4, C 2
Malignant gestational trophoblastic disease	4	4
Cervical cancer awaiting treatment	I 4, C 2	I 4, C 2
Current breast cancer	1	4
Endometrial cancer	I 4, C 2	I 4, C 2
Current pelvic inflammatory disease	I 4, C 2	I 4, C 2
Some current sexually transmitted infections	I 4, C 2	I 4, C 2
Known pelvic tuberculosis	I 4, C 3	I 4, C 3

I, initiation; C, continuation; 1, no restriction; 2, advantages outweigh risks; 3, caution, risks usually outweigh advantages; 4, contraindication, unacceptable health risk.
Source: WHO. *Medical Eligibility Criteria for Contraceptive Use.* 3rd edn. Geneva: Reproductive Health and Research, World Health Organization, 2004. Also available on the web at www.who.int/reproductive-health/publications/MEC_3/mec.pdf.

Side effects

Menstrual disturbance. Copper IUDs are associated with increased menstrual bleeding and dysmenorrhea. In clinical trials, up to 15% of women discontinue for these reasons. Bleeding can be both heavier and more prolonged. In contrast, the hormone-releasing IUD decreases blood flow. After 1 year of use, median blood loss fell to 10 mL among a sample of women with menorrhagia

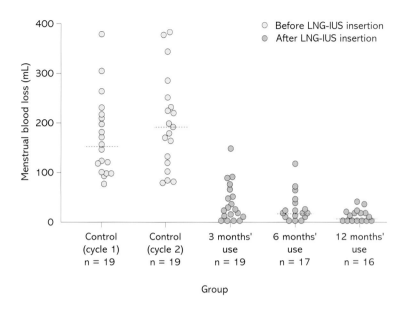

Figure 4.3 Menstrual blood loss among menorrhagic women during two control cycles before insertion of the levonorgestrel-releasing intrauterine system (LNG-IUS) and at 3, 6 and 12 months of use. Reproduced with permission from Andersson, Rybo 1990.

(Figure 4.3). Many women experience frequent spotting during the first 3 months of use, and new users should be advised that this will happen. Women who receive good information about the method have been shown to have higher continuation rates.

Perforation of the uterus occurs in 1.3 of every 1000 insertions. It is often unnoticed. Routine follow-up 6 weeks after insertion allows most perforations to be detected. Absent threads should be investigated by ultrasound. At this stage, an IUD inside the abdominal cavity can often be retrieved laparoscopically. If left for months, local adhesion formation often necessitates removal by laparotomy. If the tails have simply been drawn up inside the cervical canal but the device is in the correct position within the uterus, it can be left in place and the user reassured that the IUD will be no less effective.

Expulsion. Reported expulsion rates vary from less than 1% to almost 10% in the first year of use. Expulsion is most common in the first 3 months. Many clinicians advise IUD users to check to feel the IUD strings regularly in order to detect expulsion. In reality, this is often not easy to do and results more often in anxiety than in the detection of unrecognized expulsion.

Ectopic pregnancy. Intrauterine contraception is much more effective for the prevention of intrauterine pregnancy than it is for the prevention of ectopic pregnancy. If pregnancy occurs with an IUD in the uterus, the risk of ectopic pregnancy is around 3–5% (< 1% for the levonorgestrel IUS). The risk of an ectopic pregnancy without an IUD in the uterus is approximately 1.9% in the USA and UK. However, as failure is uncommon, the overall risk of ectopic pregnancy with the copper IUD is less than 1.5 per 1000 woman-years of IUD use.

Pelvic infection. The risk of pelvic infection associated with IUD use has been overestimated. A meta-analysis undertaken by the WHO in 1992 suggested that the risk had halved during the 1980s, presumably because providers are more aware of the association and avoid IUD insertion in women at increased risk of infection. Infection is most likely to occur during the 20 days following insertion. Thereafter, the risk of developing infection is not significantly higher than that among women using no contraception (< 1.5 per 1000 woman-years).

The risk can be reduced by using aseptic techniques during insertion and by restricting the method to women who do not have multiple partners and whose partners do not have multiple partners. When the prevalence of sexually transmitted infection is high, screening, especially for *Chlamydia*, is recommended prior to insertion. According to the WHO *Selected Practice Recommendations*, prophylactic broad-spectrum antibiotics are not generally recommended for IUD insertion, but may be considered in settings in which high prevalence of STIs is combined with limited STI screening.

If a woman using an IUD is diagnosed with pelvic inflammatory disease, she should be treated with the appropriate antibiotics. There is no need to remove the IUD if she wishes to continue using the method; however, if she does not wish to keep the IUD, it should not be removed until after antibiotics have been started.

Insertion and removal

For women who are using effective contraception (including abstinence), an IUD can be inserted at any time in the cycle. Otherwise, insertion should be limited to the first 7 days of the cycle. Postpartum insertion should be delayed until 6 weeks after childbirth, when the risk of expulsion is lower and, in women who are lactating, the risk of perforation will have returned to normal. An IUD can be inserted immediately after spontaneous or therapeutic abortion, although expulsion rates may be higher after second-trimester abortions. IUDs specifically designed for immediate postpartum insertion are being developed.

Unless pregnancy is desired, removal should be undertaken only in the late luteal phase of the cycle or in the first 7 days. In menopausal women, the IUD should be left for 1 year after the last menstrual period. If the IUD threads are not visible or snap during removal, it may be possible to remove the device with a specially designed hook or a pair of artery forceps.

If conception occurs with an IUD in place there is an increased risk of second-trimester miscarriage, premature delivery and infection. If the woman wishes to continue the pregnancy and if the strings of the IUD are visible or if it can be retrieved safely from the cervical canal, the device should be removed. If removal is not possible it should be left in place. If termination of pregnancy is desired, the IUD can be removed at the time of the abortion.

Non-contraceptive benefits

Popularity of the LNG-IUS is increasing in the UK, where the Mirena system now accounts for some 10% of hormonal contraceptive use. It is likely that the associated amenorrhea adds to the acceptability of this long-acting method of contraception.

In most of Europe, including the UK, this IUS is also licensed for the management of menorrhagia. A slightly smaller device is likely to be licensed in the UK by 2006 for hormone replacement therapy. The IUS provides the progestogen necessary for protection against endometrial cancer. Estrogen can be given by the user's preferred route of administration and at a dose that can be titrated against symptom relief. Given recent concerns about the role of progestogens in the risk of breast cancer associated with HRT, this strategy is likely to prove popular, since the dose of progestogen is both extremely low and targeted to the endometrium.

Future prospects

For many years, scientists have been exploring the possibility of developing a tailless IUD, since it is thought that the tail, hanging down into the non-sterile vagina, increases the risk of infection. It is hard to see how a tailless device could be easily removed, and, as discussed earlier, the risks of infection have generally been overstated.

Attracted by the success of the levonorgestrel-releasing IUS, manufacturers are investigating the use of alternative progestogens in different doses. For women who find amenorrhea unacceptable, a slightly lower bioactive dose may reduce blood loss significantly without inhibiting it altogether. Of more scientific interest are efforts to find a way to overcome the 3–6 months of spotting common when women first start Mirena. Antiprogestogens and angiogenesis inhibitors have been suggested as possible candidates to be used either in combination with a progestogen or alone.

Key points – intrauterine devices and systems

- Intrauterine devices (IUDs) offer extremely safe, long-acting and highly effective contraception.
- Copper IUDs are often associated with slightly longer and heavier menstrual periods, and this is the commonest reason for discontinuation.
- The levonorgestrel-releasing intrauterine system (LNG-IUS) causes endometrial atrophy and, after a few months of spotting, is often associated with amenorrhea.
- There is an increased risk of pelvic infection at the time of IUD insertion. Women whose lifestyle puts them at risk of sexually transmitted infections should be screened before IUD insertion.
- Uterine perforation and expulsion of IUDs is unusual and related to the skill of the provider.
- The LNG-IUS can be used for the treatment of menorrhagia and to provide the progestogen component of hormone replacement therapy.

Key references

Andersson JK, Rybo G. Levonorgestrel-releasing intrauterine device in the treatment of menorrhagia. *Br J Obstet Gynaecol* 1990;97:690–4.

Chi I-C. What we have learned from recent IUD studies: a researcher's perspective. *Contraception* 1993; 48:81–108.

Doll H, Vessey M, Painter R. Return of fertility in nulliparous women after discontinuation of the intrauterine device: comparison with women discontinuing other methods of contraception. *BJOG* 2001; 108:304–14.

Fortney JA, Feldblum PJ, Raymond EG. Intrauterine devices. The optimal long-term contraceptive method? *J Reprod Med* 1999;44:269–74.

Grimes DA. Intrauterine devices and infertility: sifting through the evidence. *Lancet* 2001;358:6–7.

Grimes D. Intrauterine device and upper-genital-tract infection. *Lancet* 2000;356:1013–19.

Hubacher D. The checkered history and bright future of intrauterine contraception in the United States. *Perspect Sex Reprod Health* 2002; 34:98–103.

Hurskainen R, Teperi J, Rissanen P et al. Quality of life and cost-effectiveness of levonorgestrel-releasing intrauterine system versus hysterectomy for treatment of menorrhagia: a randomised trial. *Lancet* 2001;357:273–7.

Varila E, Wahlstrom T, Rauramo I. A 5-year follow-up study on the use of a levonorgestrel intrauterine system in women receiving hormone replacement therapy. *Fertil Steril* 2001;76:969–73.

WHO. *Intrauterine Devices. Technical and Managerial Guidelines for Services.* Geneva: World Health Organization, 1997.

Wildemeersch D, Batar D, Webb A et al. Gynefix. The frameless intrauterine implant – an update for interval, emergency and post-abortal contraception. *Br J Fam Plann* 1999;24:149–59.

Introduced in the early 1960s, the combined oral contraceptive pill has been used by about 200 million women worldwide. Around 33% of women in the UK using contraception take the combined oral contraceptive pill, while in the USA the figure is around 17%. It is not surprising that the combined pill is so popular, as it is extremely effective, is easy to use and has additional health benefits beyond contraception. Newer delivery systems for combined hormonal contraception (transdermal patch, vaginal ring, injectables) may be expected to increase in popularity in future.

Mode of action

Combined hormonal contraception acts mainly by inhibiting ovulation. Estrogen suppresses the development of ovarian follicles, while the progestogen (a progestin, or synthetic progesterone) inhibits the development of the LH surge and therefore ovulation. Figure 5.1 shows the hormone levels achieved with various delivery systems; Figure 5.2 shows the normal cycle. In some women, the 7-day pill-free interval (PFI) is long enough to allow follicle growth; if the interval is extended beyond 7 days, these follicles will continue to develop and, even if the woman starts taking the pill again, ovulation may occur. For women who appear to have conceived as a result of a genuine pill failure (rather than as a result of an error in taking the pill) and who wish to continue using the combined oral contraceptive, the PFI can be shortened to 4 or 5 days. In the USA, a formulation called Mircette is now available, which consists of 20 μg ethinyl estradiol and 150 μg desogestrel taken for 21 days followed by 2 days of placebo and then 5 days of 10 μg ethinyl estradiol only. The product is designed to appeal to women wishing to take the lowest possible dose of estrogen without compromising efficacy or cycle control.

   Use of combined oral contraceptives is also associated with the development of hostile cervical mucus and an atrophic

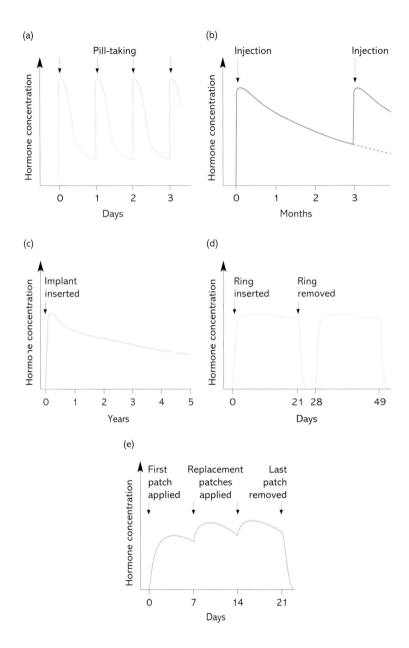

Figure 5.1 Theoretical hormone-release profiles for: (a) the oral contraceptive pill; (b) 3-monthly injections; (c) an implant; (d) vaginal rings; (e) patches.

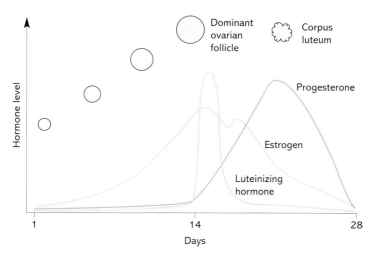

Figure 5.2 Hormone levels and follicle growth in the normal cycle.

endometrium, so that sperm transport and implantation may be impaired.

Oral preparations

The combined pill contains estrogen – usually ethinyl estradiol – and a progestogen. The estrogen dose varies from 15 to 50 µg. As the cardiovascular risks of the pill are considered to be mainly due to estrogen, preparations containing 50 µg ethinyl estradiol are reserved for special situations (see page 57). The lower the dose of estrogen, the higher the chance of poor cycle control, breakthrough bleeding and pregnancy if use is imperfect. For these reasons, most women now use pills containing 30–35 µg ethinyl estradiol.

The progestogens used in currently available pills fall broadly into three groups:
• first-generation (e.g. norethindrone)
• second-generation (e.g. levonorgestrel)
• third-generation (e.g. gestodene, desogestrel and norgestimate).
In 2001 Yasmin, a pill containing a new progestogen, drospirenone, was introduced in both Europe and the USA, but not Canada. Drospirenone has both antiandrogenic and antimineralocorticoid properties, and is said to be associated with a lower incidence of

fluid retention and 'bloating'. The manufacturers do not describe drospirenone as a fourth-generation progestogen.

Different progestogens have different potencies, and thus contraceptive efficacy is achieved at different doses.

Regimens. The pill is taken for 21 days followed by a 7-day break (the PFI), during which time withdrawal bleeding usually occurs. In the USA, most women take every-day preparations, in which inactive tablets are taken for the 7 days of the PFI. This is thought to make pill-taking less complicated.

Combined pills are available in monophasic preparations, in which every pill in the packet contains the same dose of steroids, and biphasic and triphasic preparations, where the amounts of both estrogen and progestogen change once or twice during the 21 days. There is no evidence for better cycle control with bi- or triphasic pills, and some women find these phasic preparations somewhat confusing, particularly if they want to run packets of pills together to postpone menstruation.

In the UK and the Netherlands, so-called tricycling of the pill has been common for more than 20 years; it can be achieved simply by running existing 21-day pill packets together without a break. A three-month combined pill (Seasonale) has now been licensed in the USA. It comprises 84 days of active tablets followed by 7 days of placebo, and is designed to give women only four bleeding episodes each year.

Efficacy. When the combined pill is used perfectly, the failure rate is 0.1% (1 pregnancy in 1000 women taking the pill in the first year of use). Typical use is associated with a failure rate of 8%.

New delivery systems for combined hormonal contraception

Three new combined hormonal contraceptives have come onto the market in the last few years, a once-monthly injectable regimen, a vaginal ring and a transdermal patch. Like the combined pill, all three methods work primarily by inhibiting ovulation, and all have similar side effects. The health risks and benefits are also likely to be the same as those of the combined pill, but there are as yet very few data on safety other than those considered essential before a license can be granted. Constant circulating hormone concentrations may reduce the incidence of minor side effects when compared with oral administration (see Figure 5.1). Non-oral routes of administration avoid the first-pass hepatic metabolism, allowing lower doses of steroids to be used. In theory, then, the risk of VTE, for example, associated with these delivery systems may be less than that for the oral route, but only time – and postmarketing surveillance – will tell.

Although superficially different from the combined pill, none of these new methods is radically different. They do, however, offer additional choices for women wanting a hormonal method, and would be particularly useful for the small number of women who experience nausea with the combined pill or who have chronic inflammatory bowel disease, which may be exacerbated by the oral administration of contraceptive steroids.

Combined injectable contraception. A monthly contraceptive injection, Lunelle, was licensed for use in the USA in 2002. The controlled-release preparation contains medroxyprogesterone acetate, 25 mg, and a natural estrogen ester, estradiol cypionate, 5 mg. The failure rate is around 3 pregnancies per 1000 women in the first 12 months of use. In a recent trial in the USA, no pregnancies occurred among 782 women using the method for 13 cycles of treatment. The return to fertility when the injections are stopped is rapid, which is not the case with the progestogen-only injectable (Depo-Provera). Most women establish a regular bleeding pattern, with one withdrawal bleed lasting 6 days occurring every 28 days (slightly more days of bleeding than among combined pill users). At the time of going to press, Lunelle is unavailable in the USA owing to manufacturing problems.

Transdermal contraceptive patch. A 20 cm^2 matrix patch delivering norelgestromin, 150 µg, and ethinyl estradiol, 20 µg, daily into the systemic circulation (Ortho Evra, Evra) was launched in the USA in 2002 and in the UK in 2003, and is now available elsewhere in Europe and in Canada. It is worn for 7 days for 3 consecutive weeks, followed by a patch-free interval; in a trial of 812 women using the patch for 13 cycles the overall failure rate was 1.24, and the failure rate among perfect users was 0.99/100 woman-years. Bleeding patterns are not significantly different from those associated with the combined pill, but breast discomfort and dysmenorrhea appear to be slightly more common.

Combined contraceptive vaginal ring. A flexible, soft, transparent ring (NuvaRing), with an outer diameter of 54 mm and a cross-section of 4 mm, that releases etonogestrel, 120 µg/day, and ethinyl estradiol, 15 µg/day, into the vagina came onto the market in the USA in 2002. Already licensed elsewhere in Europe, it is likely to become available in the UK in 2005. The ring is worn for 21 days and removed for 7, during which time a withdrawal bleed occurs. In a study involving over 1100 women using the ring for 13 cycles the total failure rate was 0.65 pregnancies per 100 woman-years. Cycle control is excellent, with unscheduled bleeding occurring in only 6.4% of cycles. Insertion and removal of the ring is easy, and it does not need to fit in any special place in the vagina.

Contraindications
Category 4 conditions in the WHO *Medical Eligibility Criteria* are listed in Table 5.1, and relative contraindications (category 3 conditions) in Table 5.2.

Women with hyperprolactinemia wishing to avoid pregnancy should be advised to use progestogen-only contraception; estrogen stimulates the lactotrophs, increasing prolactin concentration.

Risks and side effects
Most side effects are minor, but often lead to discontinuation. Mood change, weight gain or fluid retention, nausea and vomiting, headache, chloasma, loss of libido, mastalgia and breast enlargement, and greasy skin are all quite common complaints

TABLE 5.1

WHO *Medical Eligibility Criteria* 2004 category 4 conditions (absolute contraindications) for use of the combined oral contraceptive pill

- Breastfeeding < 6 weeks postpartum
- Smoking ≥ 15 cigarettes/day and age ≥ 35
- Multiple risk factors for cardiovascular disease
- Hypertension: systolic pressure ≥ 160 or diastolic ≥ 100 mmHg
- Hypertension with vascular disease
- Current or history of deep-vein thrombosis/pulmonary embolism
- Major surgery with prolonged immobilization
- Known thrombogenic mutations
- Current or history of ischemic heart disease
- Current or history of stroke
- Complicated valvular heart disease
- Migraine with aura
- Migraine without aura and age ≥ 35 (continuation)
- Current breast cancer
- Diabetes for ≥ 20 years or with severe vascular disease or with severe nephropathy, retinopathy or neuropathy
- Active viral hepatitis
- Severe cirrhosis
- Benign or malignant liver tumors

Source: WHO. *Medical Eligibility Criteria for Contraceptive Use.* 3rd edn. Geneva: Reproductive Health and Research, World Health Organization, 2004. Also available on the web at www.who.int/reproductive-health/publications/MEC_3/mec.pdf.

among pill users. Many improve or disappear within 3–6 months of starting the pill; this information may be helpful to women considering changing their method of contraception because of side effects. As some side effects may be alleviated by changing the estrogen dose or type of progestogen, it is worth trying an alternative if time alone does not solve the problem.

TABLE 5.2

WHO *Medical Eligibility Criteria* 2004 category 3 conditions (relative contraindications) for use of the combined oral contraceptive pill

- Multiple risk factors for arterial disease
- Hypertension: systolic blood pressure 140–159 or diastolic pressure 90–99 mmHg, or adequately treated to below 140/90 mmHg
- Some known hyperlipidemias
- Diabetes mellitus with vascular disease
- Smoking (< 15 cigarettes/day) and age ≥ 35 years
- Obesity
- Migraine, even without aura, and age ≥ 35 years
- Breast cancer with > 5 years without recurrence
- Breastfeeding until 6 months postpartum
- Postpartum and not breastfeeding until 21 days after childbirth
- Current or medically treated gallbladder disease
- History of cholestasis related to combined oral contraceptives
- Mild cirrhosis
- Taking rifampicin (rifampin) or certain anticonvulsants

Source: WHO. *Medical Eligibility Criteria for Contraceptive Use.* 3rd edn. Geneva: Reproductive Health and Research, World Health Organization, 2004. Also available on the web at www.who.int/reproductive-health/publications/MEC_3/mec.pdf.

Serious side effects mainly involve the cardiovascular system; the pill affects both venous and arterial circulation. Although the combined pill is associated with alterations in lipids and triglycerides, it is thought that the cardiovascular side effects (both venous and arterial) result from the increased tendency of the blood to clot.

Myocardial infarction (MI) is rare among women of reproductive age. There is almost no increase in the risk of MI among normotensive women who use combined oral contraceptives, regardless of age. However, hypertension among pill users increases the risk of MI by at least three times, and diabetes increases the risk by an unknown amount. Smoking greatly increases the risk of MI. The relative risk of MI in heavy smokers who use combined oral contraceptives may be as high as ten times that of smokers who do not take the pill.

The risk of MI is unaffected by the duration of use of combined oral contraceptives, and after use is ended it returns to that of women who have never used this form of contraception (see below, in the section on stroke).

Stroke. Ischemic stroke is also very rare in women of reproductive age. Among normotensive women who do not smoke, pill use increases the relative risk of ischemic stroke by about 1.5, but the absolute risk remains extremely small. The risk is increased by hypertension (threefold) and by smoking (two- to threefold).

The risk of hemorrhagic stroke is not increased in normotensive women under 35 years of age who do not smoke. However, the incidence of hemorrhagic stroke increases with age, and this effect is magnified by use of the combined oral contraceptive. Hypertension increases the risk by a factor of around ten, and smoking by about three times.

The risks of MI and stroke are not affected by the duration of use of combined oral contraceptives, and women who have used this form of contraception in the past are not at increased risk for either condition. There is insufficient evidence to prove that the type of progestogen used influences the risk of either stroke or MI.

Venous thromboembolism. Current users of the combined oral contraceptive pill have an increased risk of VTE three to six times that of non-users. The absolute risk is small and much less than that conferred by pregnancy (Table 5.3). The risk probably declines after the first year of use but persists until use of the pill is stopped, when the risk rapidly falls to that of non-users. The risk of VTE is not increased by either smoking or hypertension. However, pills that contain either desogestrel or gestodene probably carry a

TABLE 5.3

Incidence of venous thromboembolism per 100 000 women

Never used hormonal contraception	5
Current users: levonorgestrel	15
Current users: desogestrel/gestodene	25–30
Pregnancy	60

small risk of VTE beyond that attributable to pills that contain levonorgestrel. The so-called 'third-generation pill scare' of 1995 has made many doctors nervous of prescribing new brands of combined pills (such as Yasmin) for fear of an as yet unrecognized increased risk of VTE.

Breast cancer. Many women taking the combined oral contraceptive pill worry about breast cancer. Published data are difficult to interpret because pill formulations and patterns of reproduction (particularly age at first pregnancy) have changed with time.

A large meta-analysis of most of the published data suggested in 1996 that use of the combined oral contraceptive pill *is* associated with an increase in the risk of having breast cancer diagnosed. The risk does not seem to be affected by the dose or type of estrogen or progestogen taken, neither is it influenced by the duration of use. After 1 year of pill use, the relative risk of breast cancer is increased to 1.24, and it does not rise beyond that figure whether the woman continues to take the pill for 5, 10 or 20 years. The risk of metastases, however, seems to be lower than that in women who have not used the pill. The increased risk declines when the pill is stopped, but does not return to that of non-users until 10 years after stopping. The risk for women with a family history of breast cancer or a personal history of benign breast disease does not appear to be increased more than that for women without a personal or family history.

A more recent case-control study from the USA that involved more than 4500 women with breast cancer suggested no increase in the risk of breast cancer among ever-users of the combined pill. However, the confidence intervals in this study were similar to those of the much larger meta-analysis.

The exact relationship between the combined pill and breast cancer is still not fully understood. If there is an association, it is possible that pill use results in the earlier detection of tumors, or that there is late-stage promotion of the disease.

Cervical cancer. Data on the risk of cervical cancer among pill users are also difficult to interpret, as barrier methods confer some protection and the etiology of cervical cancer is linked to sexual activity. Adenocarcinoma of the cervix is rare, but its risk does appear to increase twofold among women using the combined pill. Recently published data have suggested as much as a fourfold increase in the risk of squamous carcinoma of the cervix among women with persistent human papilloma virus (HPV) infection who have used the pill for more than 5 years. However, pill users are a captive population for cervical screening, facilitating early detection and treatment, and almost all squamous carcinoma of the cervix should be preventable, particularly if screening for HPV becomes routine and vaccination against cervical cancer becomes available.

Benign hepatic adenoma is a rare consequence of combined oral contraceptive use.

Non-contraceptive benefits

Combined oral contraceptives confer a number of health benefits. Most women find that their menstrual periods are lighter, shorter and more regular during pill use. Periods also tend to be less painful and premenstrual symptoms less troublesome. The combined pill is often the first choice of treatment for menorrhagia, dysmenorrhea, premenstrual syndrome and anovulatory dysfunctional uterine bleeding. Other benefits include a decreased incidence (during pill use) of benign breast lumps, functional ovarian cysts, endometriosis, possibly pelvic inflammatory disease and certainly acne.

When hormonal contraception is being used for the management of a medical problem the risk–benefit balance changes somewhat and the WHO *Medical Eligibility Criteria* may be less appropriate.

This method of contraception protects against both ovarian and endometrial cancer. Use of the combined pill for 5 years reduces the risk of epithelial ovarian cancer by 50% and the effect lasts for at least 10 years after use has stopped. Similarly, the risk of endometrial cancer declines by 20% after 1 year and by about 50% after 4 years of use. The protective effect lasts for perhaps as long as 15 years after stopping the pill.

Practical prescribing

A full history should be taken to exclude risk factors that might contraindicate combined hormonal contraception or suggest the need for further investigation. Blood pressure should be measured, and it may be helpful to record baseline weight. Pelvic examination is not routinely indicated at the first visit unless there is reason to suspect gynecological pathology. Women do not like pelvic examinations and some, particularly the young, may be deterred from starting or continuing with the method if examination is seen as a necessary prerequisite. In the *Selected Practice Recommendations for Contraceptive Use*, the WHO recommends that the measurement of blood pressure is the only test that should be mandatory before use of combined hormonal contraception is started. Other tests, including cholesterol measurement and cervical smear, which are more likely to be done in the USA than in the UK, are not considered to contribute substantially to the safe and effective use of the method.

Cervical smears should be carried out in accordance with national policy. A baseline breast examination is sometimes recommended in new users over the age of 35 years, but is not essential. Screening for abnormal lipid or coagulation profiles is necessary only for women with risk factors.

New users should start with a low-dose pill (30–35 μg estrogen). Breakthrough bleeding usually settles within the first 3 months, but if it persists, and after gynecologic causes have been excluded, a higher-dose pill or one containing a different type of progestogen may be tried. Women on long-term enzyme-inducing drugs, such as some anticonvulsants, griseofulvin or rifampicin (rifampin), should use a 50 μg estrogen preparation to ensure optimal efficacy; alternatively, a standard regimen of combined injectable contraception, which provides a relatively high dose, can be used.

It has become common practice to advise women taking broad-spectrum antibiotics that the efficacy of their combined oral contraceptive may be reduced. While the evidence for any effect is poor, there are insufficient data to recommend abandoning this practice. It is not sensible to change these women to a high-dose pill, as most courses of antibiotics are taken for less than 2 weeks. Women should be advised to continue taking the pill but to use secondary protection (condoms) or abstain from penetrative sex for the duration of antibiotic use and 7 days thereafter. For women taking prolonged courses of antibiotics, such as tetracyclines for acne, 2 weeks of secondary protection after completion of the course is sufficient to allow the resumption of normal pill efficacy. Data for interactions between antibiotics and combined hormonal injections, patches and rings are lacking.

Women should be carefully instructed about taking the pill and what to do when pills are forgotten (Figure 5.3 and Figure 5.4).

No combined hormonal contraceptive offers protection against HIV infection and other STIs, and this should be made clear to users.

Having a break from using the pill for a few months has no effect on the risk of breast cancer, and while the cardiovascular risks decline when the pill is stopped, they recur as soon as it is started again. Unplanned pregnancies commonly occur during such breaks – most women who stop taking the pill regain normal fertility within 3 months. Prolonged amenorrhea is almost always the result of abnormalities present before the pill was started, such as polycystic ovary syndrome. There is no evidence of any adverse effect on the fetus resulting from previous pill use. If conception occurs during pill use, the risk of teratogenesis is small or non-existent.

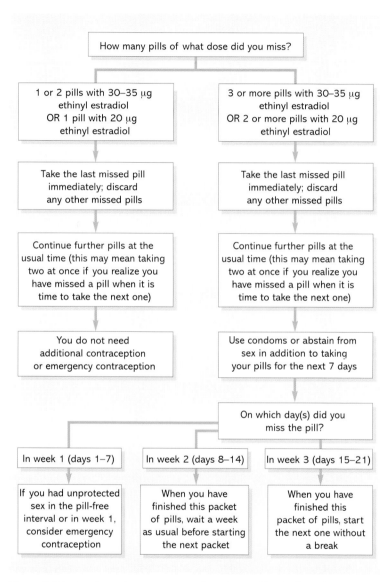

Figure 5.3 Instructions given to women who miss combined pills in the UK.

Future prospects

With the exception of implants, potential practical routes of administration for combined hormonal contraception have now been exhausted. The pharmaceutical industry will continue to

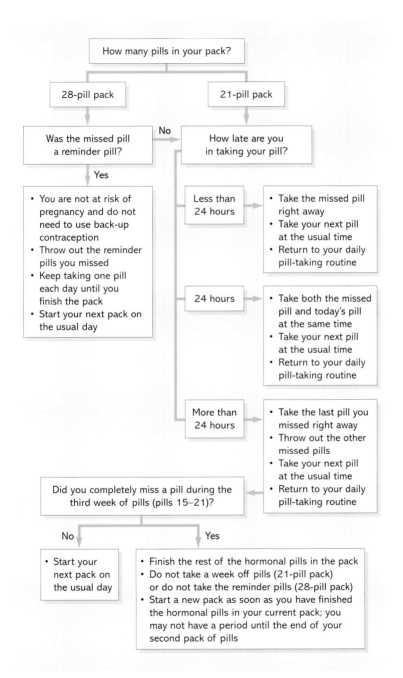

Figure 5.4 Instructions given to women who miss combined pills in the USA.

develop new progestins and, probably, to experiment with natural estrogens for contraceptive purposes. It is difficult to see how the existing methods could be improved in any way that would be clinically significant. However small the risks of cardiovascular disease and breast cancer, they deter many women from using combined hormonal methods and limit their use to women without contraindications to estrogen. The development of selective hormone-receptor modulators that bind to some tissue receptors (in the brain, ovary and uterus) but not to others (in the breast or blood vessels) will, one hopes, lead eventually to highly effective

---

Key points – combined hormonal contraception

- Combined hormonal contraception is now available via oral (pills), transdermal (patches), injectable and vaginal (rings) routes of administration.
- Failure rates are similar for all methods, at around 1 per 1000 women per year if used perfectly.
- Combined hormonal contraception increases the risk of venous thromboembolism three- to sixfold and slightly increases the risk of stroke, but is not associated with an increased risk of myocardial infarction in non-smoking, normotensive women. The absolute risk of these conditions is extremely small.
- The combined pill (and probably other combined methods) increases the risk of breast cancer by 24%.
- The risk of carcinoma of the cervix is increased fourfold, but only in women who take the pill for over 5 years *and* have persistent human papillomavirus infection.
- Since the pill requires correct and consistent use for its efficacy it is important that women are well informed about how to use it.
- The pill and other combined hormonal contraceptives confer health benefits beyond contraception, particularly in improving patterns of menstruation.
- The pill can be used continuously to avoid monthly withdrawal bleeds; the same probably applies to the patch and the ring.

hormonal contraceptives with all the health benefits and none of the risks.

Antihormones have been used for many years in the treatment of infertility (e.g. clomiphene, an estrogen antagonist, and gonadotropin-releasing hormone (GnRH) agonists as an adjunct to superovulation) and in the treatment and prevention of breast cancer (the antiestrogen tamoxifen). GnRH agonists and antagonists have been tested in a variety of forms as contraceptives for both men and women. They are expensive and not available orally, and their role so far is limited.

Antiprogestins (antiprogesterones) have been tested as daily, once-weekly and once-monthly pills, and are likely to prove to be highly effective contraceptives without the side effects associated with estrogen. It is also possible that they may confer some protection against breast cancer. In a trial involving over 100 women in the UK and China, a daily dose of either 2 or 5 mg mifepristone (RU486) inhibited ovulation in over 90% of women and was associated with endometrial changes unlikely to support implantation. Most women, particularly those taking 5 mg/day, were amenorrheic. Mifepristone has been shown to be highly effective as an emergency contraceptive and is marketed as such in China. The politics surrounding the use of antiprogestins (which are known to be abortifacient), particularly in the USA, have slowed their development. However, they show such promise that the interest of the pharmaceutical industry in these compounds has been rekindled.

Key references

Audet MC, Moreau M, Koltun WD et al. Evaluation of contraceptive efficacy and cycle control of a transdermal contraceptive patch vs an oral contraceptive. *JAMA* 2001;285:2347–54.

Baird DT, Glasier AF. Contraception. *BMJ* 1999;319:969–72.

Beral V, Hermon C, Kay C et al. Mortality associated with oral contraceptive use: 25-year follow-up of a cohort of 46 000 women from the Royal College of General Practitioners' oral contraception study. *BMJ* 1999;318:96–100.

Brown A, Cheng L, Lin S, Baird DT. Daily low-dose mifepristone has contraceptive potential by suppressing ovulation and menstruation: A double-blind randomized control trial of 2 and 5 mg per day for 120 days. *J Clin Endocrinol Metab* 2002;87:63–70.

The Collaborative Group on Hormonal Factors in Breast Cancer. Breast cancer and hormonal contraceptives: a collaborative re-analysis of individual data on 53 297 women with breast cancer and 100 239 women without breast cancer from 54 epidemiological studies. *Lancet* 1996;347:1713–27.

Dunn N, Thorogood M, Faragher B et al. Oral contraceptives and myocardial infarction: results of the MICA case-control study. *BMJ* 1999;318:1579–83.

Kaunitz AM. Lunelle™ monthly injectable contraceptive. An effective, safe and convenient new birth control option. *Arch Gynecol Obstet* 2001;265:119–23.

Marchbanks PA, McDonald JA, Wilson HG et al. Oral contraceptives and the risk of breast cancer. *N Engl J Med* 2002;346:2025–32.

Moreno V, Bosch FX, Muñoz N et al. International Agency for Research on Cancer (IARC) Multicentric Cervical Cancer Study Group. Effect of oral contraceptives on risk of cervical cancer in women with human papillomavirus infection: the IARC multicentric case-control study. *Lancet* 2002;359:1085–92.

Roumen FJME, Apter D, Mulders TMT, Dieben TOM. Efficacy, tolerability and acceptability of a novel contraceptive vaginal ring releasing etonogestrel and ethinyl oestradiol. *Hum Reprod* 2001; 16:469–75.

Tanis BC, van den Bosch MAAJ, Kemmeren JM et al. Oral contraceptives and the risk of myocardial infarction. *N Engl J Med* 2001;345:1787–93.

Truitt ST, Fraser AB, Grimes DA et al. Hormonal contraception during lactation. A systematic review of randomized controlled trials. *Contraception* 2003;68:233–8.

WHO. *Cardiovascular Disease and Steroid Hormone Contraception.* WHO Technical Report Series No. 877. Geneva: World Health Organization, 1998.

WHO. *Improving Access to Quality Care in Family Planning. Selected Practice Recommendations for Contraceptive Use. 2nd edn.* Geneva: Reproductive Health and Research, World Health Organization, 2004. Also available on the web at www.who.int/reproductive-health/publications/rhr_02_7/spr.pdf.

6 Progestogen-only methods

Progestogen-only hormonal methods include pills (also known as minipills), injections, implants and intrauterine delivery systems (the last are covered in Chapter 4). These contraceptives protect against pregnancy by:

- thickening cervical mucus, thus hindering sperm motility
- suppressing ovulation (depending on the progestogen used and the dose)
- slowing ovum transport through the fallopian tubes
- rendering the endometrium inhospitable to fertilized ova.

Progestogen-only methods are thought to be safer than estrogen-containing contraceptives, since it is estrogen in the combined pill that has been associated with thrombotic events. As with combined oral contraceptives, no progestogen-only contraceptive offers protection against HIV infection and other STIs, and this should be made clear to users.

Progestogen may be less effective if used in combination with drugs that induce liver enzymes, such as barbiturates, rifampicin (rifampin) and griseofulvin. Unlike estrogen-containing contraceptives, progestogen-only methods do not reduce breast milk quantity. Progestogens are secreted into breast milk in variable amounts, but this has not been found to have negative effects on babies, in contrast to the case for the combined pill.

Progestogen-only pills

Oral contraceptives containing only low doses of norgestrel, norethisterone or norethindrone (and, in the UK, levonorgestrel, desogestrel and etynodiol diacetate) have failure rates ranging from 0.5% for perfect use to 5% for typical use. If pregnancy does occur during minipill use, the risk of ectopic pregnancy is higher than usual, possibly because progestogens slow ovum transport.

Pill-taking is started on the first day of the cycle, and a new packet is begun the day after finishing the previous one; there is no pill-free interval. The progestogen effect on the cervical mucus peaks within 2–3 hours and then gradually diminishes. The pill must be taken at the same time every day to avoid an increased risk of pregnancy. Women who have menstrual cycles (including breastfeeding women) and who have missed one or more pills by more than 3 hours should take a pill immediately and then continue taking the pills as usual, but also abstain from sex or use additional contraception for the next 2 days, and consider emergency contraception (for women who are breastfeeding and amenorrheic, and less than 6 months postpartum, no additional contraceptive protection is needed). Breakthrough bleeding is common during minipill use, since many women have irregular follicle growth and ovulation and so bleed irregularly.

Progestogen-only pill-users appear to return to normal fertility more quickly than women who use combination pills. Side effects such as depression, nausea and breast tenderness also seem less common. Because of disordered follicle growth and ovulation, persistent follicles (with ultrasound appearances of simple ovarian cysts) are common. Most of them disappear with the next menstrual bleed.

A progestogen-only pill (Cerazette) containing desogestrel, 75 µg/day, is now available in the UK, but not the USA. This pill differs from earlier forms of progestogen-only pill in that the dose of desogestrel is sufficient to inhibit ovulation in almost every cycle of use. In theory, this should make the method more effective than the older, lower-dose progestogen-only pills. It also means that the rules for missed pills in this case are the same as for the combined pill.

Depot injection

Depo-Provera (Pfizer [Pharmacia]) is an intramuscular injection of depo-medroxyprogesterone acetate, 150 mg, that protects against pregnancy for at least 3 months, with a 1–2 week grace period thereafter. In many countries, the number of women using this contraceptive rivals that using the pill. The first Depo-Provera injection is given within 7 days of the onset of menstruation to be sure that the woman is not already pregnant. The depo-medroxyprogesterone acetate acts as a timed-release depot of progestogen in the muscle. Serum concentration of medroxyprogesterone acetate rises slowly to a peak at about 3 weeks and then gradually decreases until the depot is exhausted. The method is more than 99% effective in the first year of use. Like other progestogen-only contraceptives, Depo-Provera is associated with irregular bleeding, including spotting and long periods of light bleeding. Up to 80% of women will have amenorrhea by the end of one year of use.

This type of contraceptive has a stronger inhibitory effect on ovulation than other progestogen-only methods. As a result, normal fertility does not return as quickly when it is discontinued. Women with lower bodyweights tend to become pregnant sooner. Levels of high-density lipoproteins decrease among users. Sickle-cell anemia and seizures may improve. The thick cervical mucus resulting from use may offer some protection against pelvic inflammatory disease.

Long-term use of depo-medroxyprogesterone acetate appears to result in a decrease in bone density, and it is not clear if the loss is entirely reversed after use is stopped. This question is particularly important if Depo-Provera is used by adolescents who have yet to achieve their peak bone mass. In the USA, the manufacturer, in consultation with the FDA, has added a warning about this phenomenon and states that use of the method for more than 2 years is not recommended unless other contraceptives are 'inadequate' for the woman. In the UK, the Committee on Safety of Medicines advises limiting the use of Depo-Provera as a first-line contraceptive for adolescents unless other methods are unsuitable or unacceptable; it recommends that all women should be re-evaluated after using the method for 2 years.

Implants

Norplant (Wyeth) comprises six flexible, slender capsules that are inserted under the skin, usually the inner surface of the upper arm. They can be felt, and their outline is sometimes visible. This system provides a continuous low daily dose of levonorgestrel via porous silicone tubes. Serum hormone levels are lower and more constant than with the minipill. The capsules must be removed and, if desired, replaced at the end of their effectiveness, which should be about 7 years (although the US registration remains at 5 years of use). Norplant is virtually as effective as sterilization in the first year of use, with a failure rate lower than 1%. Over a full 5-year period, the failure rate is just over 1%. Although the up-front cost for Norplant is high, when compared with the 5-year cost of other methods it is cheaper than most.

Healthcare workers who insert Norplant need special training. The six capsules are placed under the skin through a single, small, puncture-type incision of about 3 mm, using a trocar. The procedure generally takes 10–20 minutes, and local anesthetic is used. The capsules are inserted one at a time and placed so that they do not touch each other and the progestogen can diffuse easily from each implant. Because the incision is so tiny, it seldom leaves a detectable scar, but inflammation or infection at the insertion site occurs occasionally. If the capsules are inserted too deeply, they may be more difficult to remove later.

If implants are inserted during the first 7 days of the menstrual cycle, no other 'back-up' contraception is needed. If the insertion takes place at any other time during the monthly cycle, use of an additional method of contraception is recommended during the first 24 hours.

Irregular bleeding or, less commonly, amenorrhea is most likely to occur during the first year of use when circulating levonorgestrel concentrations are slightly higher. Regular menstrual periods may return as the serum progestogen level declines. Many women report a small weight gain when using Norplant, but this is usually less than that associated with injectable contraceptives. Fertility returns almost immediately after the capsules are removed.

Removal can be more difficult and more uncomfortable than insertion. The incision for removal may need to be longer than the original. Because they are visible on radiographs or ultrasound scans, the capsules are easily located, even if they cannot be felt.

On rare occasions, a second visit is needed to remove all the capsules.

In the UK, adverse publicity concerning the possible side effects of Norplant resulted in a reduction in demand, and the product was withdrawn from sale by the distributors, Hoechst Marion Roussel, in October 1999. In the USA, Norplant was recalled in 2000 because of concerns that certain lots of the plastic tubing would not allow for adequate delivery of the contraceptive steroid. In fact, this proved not to be the case. Nonetheless, the manufacturer, Wyeth Pharmaceuticals, decided not to reintroduce the method to the US market and offered to pay for removals in 2002. Thus, although still licensed in the USA at the time of going to press, the method is no longer available there.

Implanon, an implant manufactured by Organon Laboratories, is currently available in the UK and elsewhere in Europe, but not yet in the USA. It is expected to be launched in the USA in 2005.

Implanon contains etonogestrel, a progestogen that is less androgenic than levonorgestrel. It consists of a single implant with a disposable inserter (Figure 6.1), making it easier to insert and remove than Norplant. The implant lasts for 3 years, and the dose of etonogestrel is sufficient to prevent ovulation in everyone who uses it, so that in theory it may be associated with amenorrhea a little more often than Norplant. A very small number of pregnancies has been reported during 3 years of Implanon use. Most seem to arise from incorrect implant insertion or because the woman is already pregnant at the time of insertion. In all other respects, Implanon is very similar to Norplant.

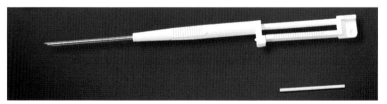

Figure 6.1 The single-rod contraceptive implant Implanon, shown with its disposable inserter.

Key points – progestogen-only methods

- Progestogen-only methods are available in many formulations, including pills, injections and subdermal implants.
- Progestogen-only methods probably work by several mechanisms, including suppression of ovulation.
- It is thought that progestogen-only methods may be safer than combined hormonal methods, because they do not contain estrogen.
- Lactating women who choose hormonal contraception should use progestogen-only rather than combined hormonal methods.
- Classical progestogen-only pills are more likely than combined pills to allow ovulation (and hence pregnancy) if a pill is skipped or not taken at the right time.
- A desogestrel-only pill is available in the UK. The dose is sufficient to inhibit ovulation in every cycle, and the missed-pill procedure is the same as for the combined pill.
- Irregular bleeding and amenorrhea are the most notable side effects of progestogen-only methods.

Contraindications

Although many regulatory agencies insist that labeled contraindications be the same for progestogen-only and combined pills, the WHO *Medical Eligibility Criteria* clearly list fewer higher-order contraindications and cautions for progestogen-only pills. In fact, the only category 4 contraindication is current cancer (especially breast cancer), listed for all progestogen-only methods: pills, implants and injections.

There are several category 3 relative contraindications, some of which vary by specific method and by whether the method is being initiated or continued. Category 3 relative contraindications for these methods are listed in Table 6.1.

Those contraindications that apply to injections only are classified as category 3 because of the much higher dose of progestogen in injectable contraceptives.

TABLE 6.1

WHO *Medical Eligibility Criteria* 2004 category 3 conditions (relative contraindications) for use of progestogen-only methods

- Breastfeeding at less than 6 weeks postpartum (all methods)
- Current deep-vein thrombosis or pulmonary embolism (all methods)
- Previous breast cancer with no evidence of disease for 5 years (all methods)
- Active viral hepatitis (all methods)
- Severe decompensated cirrhosis (all methods)
- Benign hepatic adenoma (all methods)
- Malignant hepatoma (all methods)
- Current or history of ischemic heart disease or stroke (injections, starting or continuing; continuation of pills or implants)
- Migraine with aura (continuation of all progestogen-only methods)
- Unexplained vaginal bleeding (injections and implants)
- Use of certain drugs: rifampicin (rifampin), griseofulvin, phenytoin, carbamazepine, barbiturates, primidone (pills; implants)
- Multiple risk factors for arterial cardiovascular disease (injections only)
- Systolic blood pressure > 160 or diastolic > 100 mmHg (injections only)
- Vascular disease (injections only)
- Diabetes with nephropathy, other vascular disease or disease duration of > 20 years (injections only)

Source: WHO. *Medical Eligibility Criteria for Contraceptive Use*. 3rd edn. Geneva: Reproductive Health and Research, World Health Organization, 2004. Also available on the web at www.who.int/reproductive-health/publications/MEC_3/mec.pdf.

Risks and side effects

An erratic bleeding pattern is the most notable side effect and is common to all progestogen-only methods. However, total blood loss is usually less than with normal menses. If regular periods are important to a woman, progestogen-only methods may not be a good choice.

It is not unusual for women to report weight gain while using a progestogen-only method of contraception. Fluid retention may also occur, and some women note an increase in the number or intensity of headaches, mood changes, acne or breast tenderness. These reactions may disappear or diminish after several months of use.

Further side effects are noted under the individual formulation types.

Future prospects

Implants using other progestins, such as Nestorone, are in the pipeline, although it is unlikely that they will be substantially different from Norplant or Implanon. It is unclear how they will be received in the UK and the USA, where other implants do not seem to be able to stay on the market long, owing to adverse publicity, liability issues and low demand.

Work continues on the development of a progestogen-only vaginal ring, which would have the same advantages as the combined vaginal ring in terms of constant release rate and less daily initiative by the woman required for effectiveness, but would otherwise be like the minipill in its mode of action, side effects and contraindications.

The manufacturers of Depo-Provera have produced a micronized version of the drug, to be called DMPA-SC, that is given subcutaneously and could therefore be self-administered so that women would not have to visit a provider every 3 months. The dose is lower (104 mg), and the method seems to be associated with a lower incidence of amenorrhea. The efficacy of DMPA-SC and the delay in return to fertility after it is discontinued appear no different from those observed with Depo-Provera. License applications have already been made in both the USA and UK.

Key references

Baheiraei A, Ardsetani N, Ghazizadeh S. Effects of progestogen-only contraceptives on breast-feeding and infant growth. *Int J Gynaecol Obstet* 2001;74:203–5.

Brache V, Faundes A, Alvarez F. Risk–benefit effects of implantable contraceptives in women. *Expert Opin Drug Saf* 2003;2:321–32.

Croxatto HB. Mechanisms that explain the contraceptive action of progestin implants for women. *Contraception* 2002;65:21–7.

Fraser IS. The promise and performance of progestogens as contraceptives. *Reprod Fertil Dev* 2001;13:713–21.

Kennedy KL, Short RV, Tully MR. Premature introduction of progestin-only contraceptive methods during lactation. *Contraception* 1997;55: 347–50.

Meirik O. Implantable contraceptives for women. *Contraception* 2002;65: 1–2.

Mishell DR Jr. Injectable contraception. *J Reprod Med* 2002;47(9 suppl):777–9.

Ortayli N. Users' perspectives on implantable contraceptives for women. *Contraception* 2002;65: 107–11.

Porter C, Rees MC. Bleeding problems and progestogen-only contraception. *J Fam Plann Reprod Health Care* 2002;28:178–81.

Power J, Guillebaud J. Long-acting progestogen contraceptives. *Practitioner* 2002;246:332, 335-9, 341.

Rice CF, Killick SR, Dieben TOM et al. A comparison of the inhibition of ovulation achieved by desogestrel 75 micrograms and levonorgestrel 30 micrograms daily. *Hum Reprod* 1999;14:982–5.

Schiappacasse V, Diaz S, Zepeda A et al. Health and growth of infants breastfed by Norplant contraceptive implants users: a six-year follow-up study. *Contraception* 2002;66:57–65.

Sivin I. Risks and benefits, advantages and disadvantages of levonorgestrel-releasing contraceptive implants. *Drug Saf* 2003;26:303–35.

Wan LS, Stiber A, Lam LY. The levonorgestrel two-rod implant for long-acting contraception: 10 years of clinical experience. *Obstet Gynecol* 2003;102:24–6.

Westhoff C. Depot-medroxyprogesterone acetate injection (Depo-Provera): a highly effective contraceptive option with proven long-term safety. *Contraception* 2003;68:75–87.

Emergency contraception is defined as any drug or device that is used after intercourse to prevent pregnancy. It is most commonly used after unprotected intercourse or following intercourse in which a condom burst or slipped.

Yuzpe regimen (combined estrogen–progestogen)

This method, named after the Canadian doctor who first described it, consists of two doses of a combination of ethinyl estradiol, 100 μg, and levonorgestrel, 0.5 mg, given 12 hours apart. In the UK, the one proprietary preparation (Schering PC4, licensed in 1984) was withdrawn in 2001 when it was superseded by levonorgestrel alone. The regimen is still marketed in the USA as Preven Emergency Contraception Kit (Barr Laboratories), but the marketer advises that the product is no longer manufactured and is only available until current supplies run out. It is perfectly possible for women who have combined oral contraceptive pills containing levonorgestrel to make up their own emergency contraceptive. Although few data are available, it seems likely that other types of progestogen (norethisterone, desogestrel) will work in the same manner.

Levonorgestrel alone

Two doses of levonorgestrel, 0.75 mg, with the first dose taken within 72 hours of intercourse and the second 12 hours after the first, is considered to be more effective than the Yuzpe regimen (Table 7.1). As it contains no estrogen, side effects, such as nausea and vomiting, are much less common. It has become the emergency contraceptive of choice in many countries. It is marketed in the USA as Plan B (Barr Laboratories) and in the UK as Levonelle-2 (Schering). In the UK it is available from pharmacists without a doctor's prescription, but is expensive (£25). In the USA, although it is generally sold as a prescription drug, in several states it may be purchased directly from a pharmacy with no doctor's prescription.

TABLE 7.1

Expected pregnancies prevented in relation to the time of administration of emergency contraception

Time (hours) after intercourse	Levonorgestrel (%)	Yuzpe regimen (%)
< 24	95	77
24–48	85	36
48–72	58	31

Data from Task Force on Postovulatory Methods of Fertility Regulation. *Lancet* 1998;332:428–33.

The market license holder is seeking approval to market the product as an over-the-counter item throughout the USA.

Recent data from a study undertaken by the WHO have demonstrated that a single 1.5 mg dose of levonorgestrel is as effective as the two 0.75 mg doses 12 hours apart. Since this simplifies the method considerably, a single-dose regimen has been adopted in the UK, but is not expected to be taken up in the USA in the near future.

Intrauterine device

Postcoital IUD insertion is sometimes used as an alternative to hormonal emergency contraception if a woman presents more than 72 hours after intercourse. IUD insertion may be used as emergency contraception for up to 5 days after the calculated earliest day of ovulation. This method is particularly useful for those wishing to continue with an IUD long term.

Modes of action

The mechanism of action of emergency contraception is not completely understood. There is good evidence that both the Yuzpe regimen and levonorgestrel inhibit or delay ovulation. The evidence is also good that ovulation inhibition is less likely the nearer to ovulation that either drug is given. Taken 5 days before ovulation, both methods will delay or inhibit the process in most women, but taken 2 days before ovulation both methods are much less effective. Data suggesting that both the Yuzpe regimen and levonorgestrel are more effective if they are taken within 24 hours of intercourse than if taken later (Table 7.1) are consistent with this observation. For both methods, evidence to support an effect on the endometrium that might inhibit implantation is poor. However, the estimated efficacy of levonorgestrel is greater than can be explained simply by the inhibition of ovulation, so it may act elsewhere in the reproductive process. An alternative explanation is that efficacy has been overestimated, as discussed below.

The IUD is known to diminish the viability of ova, the number of sperm reaching the fallopian tube and their ability to fertilize the egg. If it is inserted after fertilization has occurred, the IUD works by inhibiting implantation.

Efficacy

This is difficult to calculate for the following reasons.

- Placebo-controlled trials have never been performed and are now considered unethical.
- Many users are of unproven fertility.
- The chance of conception with unprotected intercourse is < 30% per cycle.
- It is impossible to know precisely when, in relation to ovulation, treatment has been given.

It has become common to describe the efficacy of emergency contraception in terms of the number of potential pregnancies prevented, based on calculating the risk of pregnancy for the day of the cycle on which intercourse occurred. Taken together, accumulated data suggest that the Yuzpe regimen and levonorgestrel prevent 75–85% of expected pregnancies. The IUD is even more effective and probably prevents over 95% of pregnancies.

Contraindications

There are no absolute contraindications to emergency hormonal contraception.

The WHO *Medical Eligibility Criteria* list several conditions in category 2 (general use, but with careful follow-up): a history of severe cardiovascular complications (including thromboembolism); angina; migraine; and severe liver disease. This classification implies that emergency contraception can be provided by someone with limited clinical judgment.

Multiple exposure (more than one act of intercourse prior to seeking emergency contraception) should not be regarded as a contraindication; it falls into category 1 in the *Medical Eligibility Criteria*. Emergency hormonal contraception can be given more than once in the same cycle. The user should understand that, if she conceived despite use of the first emergency contraceptive method, a second treatment will not be effective.

As there is no evidence linking teratogenicity with emergency hormonal contraception, pregnancy is not truly a contraindication. However, if there is any possibility that a woman requesting emergency contraception is already pregnant, it makes sense to diagnose the pregnancy, as emergency contraceptive pills would be wasted and management will alter.

The IUD is not recommended for women with a history of recent pelvic inflammatory disease (although histories can often be rather vague). For women at risk of an STI (category 3), IUD insertion should be covered with a broad-spectrum antibiotic.

Side effects

Nausea and vomiting. Up to 60% of women complain of nausea, and up to 16% vomit after the Yuzpe regimen; 23% of women taking levonorgestrel alone complain of nausea. Many women feel sick with worry, of course. Nausea and vomiting may decrease correct use.

Breast tenderness. The high dose of estrogen in the Yuzpe regimen may result in breast tenderness for a day or two.

Changes in the next menstrual cycle. Almost 30% of women will experience a delay in the onset of the next menstrual period of more than 3 days. Others will menstruate early. For most women, however, menses will come at the expected time following either hormonal method of emergency contraception.

Difficult/painful IUD insertion may occur, particularly in nulliparous women. Use of local anesthesia should be considered. Provided aseptic techniques are used, there should be no increased risk of infection. The risk of perforation is the same as that associated with routine IUD use.

Clinical management

Assessment. In order to exclude an ongoing pregnancy, the date of onset and normality of the last period should be discussed. To assess the risk of pregnancy, the possible efficacy of the chosen method and the need to consider an IUD, the timing of intercourse in relation to both the stage of the cycle (Figure 7.1) and the time elapsed since intercourse took place should be determined. Most of

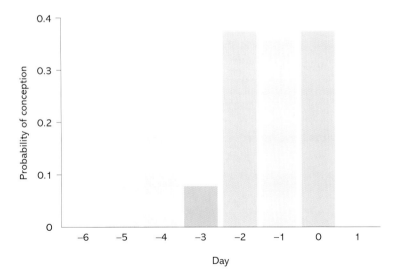

Figure 7.1 The probability of conception occurring after intercourse on the days around ovulation (day 0). Reproduced with permission from Wilcox et al. *N Engl J Med* 1995;333: 1517–21. Copyright ©1995 Massachusetts Medical Society. All rights reserved.

these questions can be answered by the woman using a self-administered questionnaire.

As there are no absolute contraindications to emergency hormonal contraception, there is really no need to measure blood pressure. A routine pelvic examination is quite unnecessary and may deter women – particularly young women – from returning for treatment in the future should the need arise. If there is any suspicion that the woman may already be pregnant, for example if the last menstrual period was abnormal in any way, it is sensible to perform a pregnancy test before treatment is given.

Counseling. Women should be informed of what is currently known about the way in which emergency contraception acts. They should also be advised of the possibility of failure. It is not necessary to ask a woman to sign a consent form before prescribing emergency contraception. Indeed, it may deter them from returning should emergency contraception ever be necessary again.

The possible side effects and the effect on the timing of the next menstrual period should be discussed. As the onset of vaginal bleeding is reassuring to women keen to avoid pregnancy, it is as well to warn about possible menstrual delay. It should be made clear to patients that emergency contraception does not work by 'bringing on a period'. Women should be advised to arrange a pregnancy test if the subsequent period does not come or if it is shorter or lighter than usual.

If the need for emergency contraception has arisen as a result of unprotected intercourse, a conventional (non-emergency) method of contraception should be discussed and, if appropriate, provided. Women who plan to use a combined hormonal method or minipill may prefer to start their pills on the first day of next menses. It is not essential to wait for the next period, but starting hormonal contraception immediately may impair recognition of a delay in menses.

Women should be encouraged to return for emergency contraception should the need arise again, and should be given information about local availability (Figure 7.2). Many women are

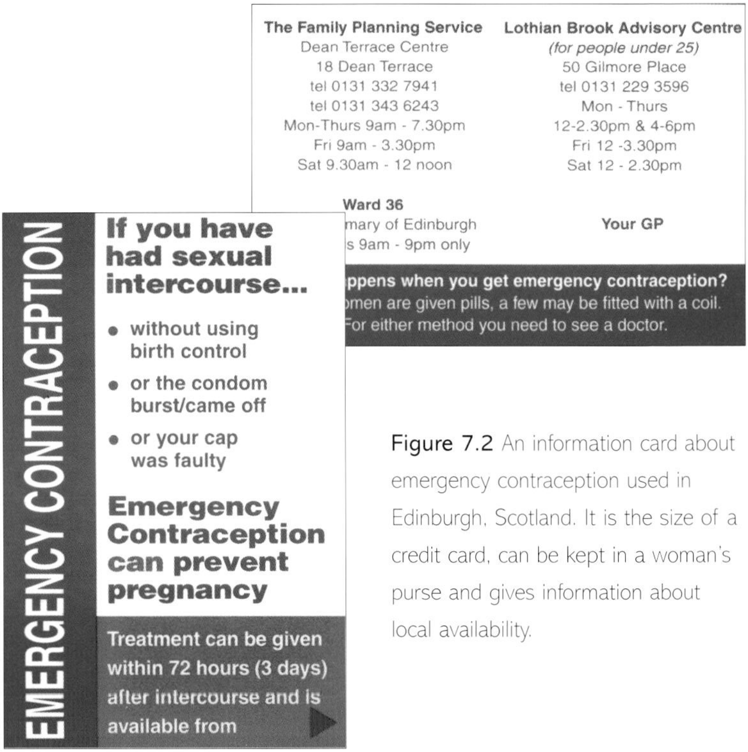

The Family Planning Service	Lothian Brook Advisory Centre
Dean Terrace Centre	(for people under 25)
18 Dean Terrace	50 Gilmore Place
tel 0131 332 7941	tel 0131 229 3596
tel 0131 343 6243	Mon - Thurs
Mon-Thurs 9am - 7.30pm	12-2.30pm & 4-6pm
Fri 9am - 3.30pm	Fri 12 -3.30pm
Sat 9.30am - 12 noon	Sat 12 - 2.30pm

Ward 36
mary of Edinburgh   Your GP
s 9am - 9pm only

ppens when you get emergency contraception?
men are given pills, a few may be fitted with a coil.
For either method you need to see a doctor.

EMERGENCY CONTRACEPTION

If you have had sexual intercourse...

- without using birth control
- or the condom burst/came off
- or your cap was faulty

Emergency Contraception can prevent pregnancy

Treatment can be given within 72 hours (3 days) after intercourse and is available from ▶

Figure 7.2 An information card about emergency contraception used in Edinburgh, Scotland. It is the size of a credit card, can be kept in a woman's purse and gives information about local availability.

embarrassed about needing emergency contraception and even more embarrassed about needing it again. It is not dangerous to use emergency contraception whenever it is required.

Concern has been expressed that making emergency contraception available off prescription results in the loss of the opportunity to discuss 'safe sex' and ongoing contraception. Most women do not need to be reminded about these issues; the very fact that they have had to use emergency contraception makes many women review their contraceptive practice. In a recent study from the UK, women under 20 and over 30 requesting emergency contraception were not at increased risk of STI (chlamydia infection) when compared with their peers who were not using emergency contraception. The prevalence of chlamydia infection was around 8% in the under-20s (all of whom should therefore be offered screening) and 1% in the over-30s. For women aged 20–30, there does seem to be an increased risk of chlamydia infection in those using emergency contraception, and they should be offered screening for infection if it is available and if it can be offered in a sensitive manner.

Advanced provision. As emergency contraception is probably more effective if used within 72 hours of intercourse, and may be more effective if used within 24 hours, it seems sensible to provide women with a supply to keep at home. A small number of trials of home use in a variety of settings have demonstrated that women are perfectly able to self-administer emergency contraception and do not tend to abandon more effective contraception.

Future prospects

Emergency contraception has become something of a holy grail in recent years, mainly because of the belief that widespread use of emergency contraception could reduce abortion rates. A number of countries have improved accessibility by taking emergency contraception off prescription and making it available without the need to see a doctor. Other strategies for increasing availability include easier access through pharmacies and, in some countries, through school nurses. These approaches are likely to become more widespread.

New methods of emergency contraception that inhibit both ovulation and implantation should prove more effective than those that inhibit ovulation only. However, nothing like this is currently in the pipeline.

The limiting factor in the effectiveness of emergency contraception may well be people's behavior, not the lack of a perfect method. It is quite clear that even those women who do know about emergency contraception, and who have easy access to it, do not use it every time there is a risk of pregnancy. The chance of conception is around 30% per cycle, so in about 70% of cases of unprotected sex, pregnancy will not result. These odds are good enough for most people to feel prepared to take a risk from time to time.

Key points – emergency contraception

- Emergency contraception can prevent pregnancy after intercourse.
- It may be more effective the sooner it is used.
- Currently available hormonal methods (levonorgestrel and the Yuzpe regimen) appear to work by inhibiting ovulation.
- A method which inhibits implantation should be more effective.
- Levonorgestrel alone is associated with few side effects, appears to be as effective as the Yuzpe regimen when taken as a single dose (1.5 mg) and is the hormonal method of choice.
- An intrauterine device is a highly effective emergency contraceptive, but insertion is invasive and requires skill.
- Limits to the effective use of emergency contraception are likely to be behavioral.
- Advance provision of emergency contraception makes sense and increases use.

Key references

Croxatto HB, Devoto L, Durand M et al. Mechanism of action of hormonal preparations used for emergency contraception: a review of the literature. *Contraception* 2001;63:111–21.

Croxatto HB, Fuentealba B, Brache V et al. Effects of the Yuzpe regimen, given during the follicular phase, on ovarian function. *Contraception* 2002;65:121–8.

Glasier A. Emergency postcoital contraception. *N Engl J Med* 1997; 337:1058–64.

Glasier A, Baird DT. The effects of self-administering emergency contraception. *N Engl J Med* 1998; 339:1–4.

Glasier A, Fairhurst K, Wyke S et al. Advanced provision of emergency contraception does not reduce abortion rates. *Contraception* 2004;69:361–6.

Kettle H, Cay S, Brown A, Glasier A. Screening for *Chlamydia trachomatis* infection is indicated for women under 30 using emergency contraception. *Contraception* 2002;66:251–3.

Task Force on Postovulatory Methods of Fertility Regulation. Comparison of three single doses of mifepristone as emergency contraception: a randomised trial. *Lancet* 1999;353:697–702.

Task Force on Postovulatory Methods of Fertility Regulation. Randomised controlled trial of levonorgestrel versus the Yuzpe regimen of combined oral contraceptives for emergency contraception. *Lancet* 1998;352:428–33.

Trussell J, Ellertson C, Dorflinger L. Effectiveness of the Yuzpe regimen of emergency contraception by cycle day of intercourse: implications for mechanism of action. *Contraception* 2003;67:167–71.

von Hertzen H, Piaggio G, Ding J et al. Low dose mifepristone and two regimens of levonorgestrel for emergency contraception: a WHO multicentre randomised trial. *Lancet* 2002;360:1803–10.

Healthy women may remain fertile until their late 40s, yet most have completed their families long before this time, and many couples choose sterilization for contraception at this point. At present, female sterilization typically involves a surgical procedure to block the fallopian tubes, thus preventing sperm from reaching an egg. Surgery has no effect on hormone production, ovulation, menstruation or sexual function. It is one of the most effective contraceptive methods, with a failure rate of less than 2% over a 10-year period. The greatest risk of failure occurs in younger women, who tend to be more sexually active and more fertile.

Sterilization surgery can be performed with a local anesthetic or under general anesthesia, most often on an outpatient or day-case basis. The procedures usually take less than 30 minutes, and most women are able to go home after an hour or two if local anesthesia is used.

Tubal occlusion does not protect against STIs, and thus, unless in a mutually monogamous relationship, couples still need a barrier method, preferably a condom.

Techniques

Female sterilization can be carried out by minilaparotomy or laparoscopy. The type of surgery depends on:
- when the procedure is done, e.g. immediately postpartum
- the health of the woman
- the preferences of the surgeon
- the medical center
- patient preference for type of procedure, incision or anesthesia.

Alternatively, the fallopian tubes can be blocked by means of the Essure device.

Minilaparotomy. If sterilization is performed immediately after childbirth, a minilaparotomy is preferred, because this approach is easiest when the uterus and tubes are high in the abdomen. Overweight women and those with adhesions from previous surgery may need a laparotomy for tubal ligation.

An incision of approximately 5 cm is made low in the abdomen, often just above the pubic hair, where it will not be very obvious. The incision is closed with a few stitches.

Laparoscopy is the approach to female sterilization most commonly used today in the USA and Europe. It is extremely safe when performed by an experienced surgeon. It is often done as an outpatient procedure, which reduces cost.

Various methods are used to block the fallopian tubes (Figure 8.1). A high-frequency electric current may be applied briefly to the narrow middle section of the fallopian tube (electrocoagulation). Scars then develop and block the tube permanently. The tubes can also be blocked by pinching them shut with mechanical devices such as metal or plastic clips or small silastic rings that are like strong rubber bands. Eventually the pinched tissue dies, forming a permanent seal. Alternatively, sutures

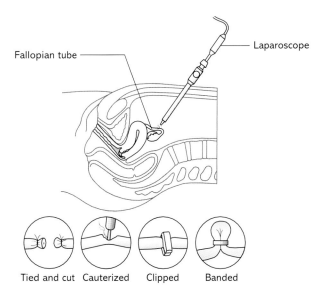

Figure 8.1 Laparoscopy and some of the tubal ligation techniques commonly used.

can be used to tie each tube, after which the surgeon removes the section of the tube between the ties.

Anesthesia. Local anesthesia is particularly appropriate for laparoscopy or minilaparotomy, because these procedures cause little trauma to the tissues and take a short time. Epidural and spinal blocks can also be used for anesthesia. General anesthesia is also effective, but can be associated with complications.

Essure, a new non-surgical system for female sterilization, was approved in the USA in November 2002 and is now also available in the European Union. Trained providers use a hysteroscope to guide insertion of a small metal coil into each fallopian tube using a thin catheter (Figure 8.2). The outpatient procedure requires no, or only local, anesthesia. The Dacron mesh embedded in the coils causes scar tissue to grow and block the tubes. This process takes 3 months to complete, and, in that interval, women must use another means of contraception. On the basis of the pivotal trial used to register this method, the manufacturers state that 92% of women can be expected to have adequate placement of the devices demonstrated on hysterosalpingogram at 3 months after insertion, and, for these women, the device should prevent over 99% of all pregnancies. Data have been reported for 2 years of use. The procedure costs somewhere in the range of US$1500–2500.

Efficacy

Sterilization is extremely effective and should be considered permanent. Occasional failures occur because an occluding device did not work properly or because electrocoagulation was not complete. A channel also can re-form in an incompletely sealed tube, allowing eggs or sperm to pass through.

Reversibility

Women should never contemplate having a tubal occlusion if there is a chance that some day they might want to have it reversed. Women under the age of 30, particularly, may be more likely to

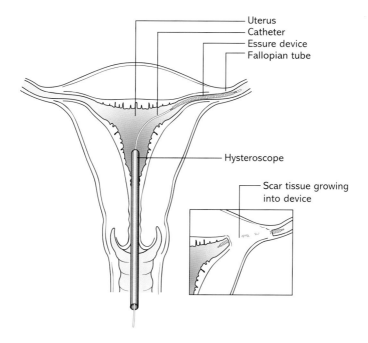

Figure 8.2 Insertion and action of the Essure device.

experience life changes, and the decision to become sterilized may be regretted. Because of this possibility, careful counseling is important before sterilization.

It is possible to repair occluded fallopian tubes so that they can function again, but this surgery is major and does not always work. Sterilization procedures that destroy too much of the tube or remove the fimbria make reversal impossible. The chances of reversing a sterilization are best if a clip or silastic band was used. Electrocoagulation causes more extensive destruction, making reversal difficult. Nothing is yet known about the reversibility of the Essure procedure, but it is likely to be very low.

Risks and possible complications

The WHO *Medical Eligibility Criteria* for female surgical sterilization deal mostly with the risks associated with surgery and general anesthesia (where used). Delay is advised when women have acute transient conditions that may make surgery more dangerous (e.g. pneumonia, STIs, eclampsia), and caution is necessary when women are suffering from chronic problems that make surgery or anesthesia more dangerous (e.g. cardiac disease, diabetes, hepatic cirrhosis). There are no criteria for the Essure procedure, since the guidelines were developed before that system became available.

Deaths resulting from female sterilization surgery are extremely rare (< 2 in 100 000); they arise mostly from complications from the use of general anesthesia. Major complications – including injuries that require further surgery to repair – occur in just under 2 out of every 1000 laparoscopy patients. The risk of complications from laparoscopy is influenced considerably by the skills of the surgeon. Clinicians who perform sterilization require special training. Furthermore, experience is important; laparoscopies performed by gynecologists who carry out fewer than 100 laparoscopies each year tend to have a much higher rate of complications.

Pregnancy following failed sterilization is associated with a higher risk of tubal pregnancy. However, 100 000 women who have had a tubal occlusion will experience fewer ectopic pregnancies than an equal number of unsterilized women who do not use contraception.

When to have a tubal occlusion

In the past, when sterilizations required hospitalization, immediately postpartum seemed a logical time to perform the procedure – the woman was already in the hospital, the surgery did not extend the hospital stay and the operation was easier. Today, however, in the USA most sterilizations are not performed in a hospital (in contrast to the UK where the majority are still performed in hospital). Many women feel that immediately after childbirth is not a good time to have any additional discomfort and pain. Tubal occlusion can also be performed immediately after an induced or spontaneous abortion, but as abortion can be an emotional, stressful event, it is not the best time for deciding on a method of contraception that is permanent. The decision to have a tubal occlusion should be made when a woman is able to think clearly about her future. Although spousal consent is not required, it is a good idea for a woman to include her partner in the decision-making process, if possible.

Future prospects

Vaccines. Political and social issues have contributed to reticence about the development of contraceptive vaccines, which are viewed by many as being too easy for governments and family-planning clinics to force on women who have few alternative choices. It is technically possible to vaccinate (at least in some species) against the egg, the sperm and the embryo. It is clearly vital, however, that a vaccine should be absolutely specific; technical problems in preventing side effects and ensuring reversibility still need to be overcome.

Key points – female sterilization

- Female sterilization is an extremely effective, safe and well-accepted way to prevent pregnancy.
- There are many techniques for female sterilization, all of them best performed by a physician with special training.
- Most sterilizations can be carried out using local anesthesia and without hospitalization.
- A non-surgical method of female sterilization (Essure) has recently been introduced in the USA.
- The timing of sterilization should be up to each woman after she has carefully considered her situation, including the wishes of her partner if she chooses to involve him.
- Sterilization should be considered permanent, because reversal, although technically possible, is costly, involves major surgery and is often not successful.

Key references

Kerin JF, Carignan CS, Cher D. The safety and effectiveness of a new hysteroscopic method for permanent birth control: results of the first Essure pbc clinical study. *Aust N Z J Obstet Gynaecol* 2001;41:364–70.

Kulier R, Boulvain M, Walker D et al. Minilaparotomy and endoscopic techniques for tubal sterilisation. *Cochrane Database Syst Rev* 2004;3:CD001328. *The Cochrane Library*, issue 4. Chichester: John Wiley & Sons, 2004 (www.thecochranelibrary.com).

Royal College of Obstetricians and Gynaecologists (RCOG). *Male and female sterilisation. Evidence-Based Clinical Guidelines No. 4.* 2nd edn. London: RCOG, 2004.

Ubeda A, Labastida R, Dexeus S. Essure: a new device for hysteroscopic tubal sterilization in an outpatient setting. *Fertil Steril* 2004; 82:196–9.

Vasectomy, the sterilization procedure for men, is simpler and safer than female sterilization and is usually performed in a doctor's surgery or clinic. A vasectomy takes only a few minutes to perform, is almost 100% effective, has few complications and is permanent. In the UK, as many men as women choose sterilization, whereas in the USA, the ratio of men to women sterilized is 1:2.5.

In a vasectomy, the two sperm ducts (vas deferens) that carry sperm from the testicles to the penis are cut. A small portion of each vas is removed, and the cut ends are closed off. A vasectomy does not influence virility, nor does it have any negative impact on overall health. The only change that takes place is that the semen contains no sperm, so it cannot cause pregnancy. Until all the sperm that were present when the surgery was performed have been ejaculated or have died, a man can still be fertile. This process takes between 2 and 4 months, or about 20 ejaculations. Another contraceptive method is needed until two consecutive specimens of semen are found to be free of sperm.

A vasectomy does not protect either partner against STIs.

Techniques

The standard vasectomy technique uses a tiny incision (Figure 9.1); the 'no-scalpel' method uses a puncture (Figure 9.2). Some incisions are so small that they need no suture. Very small forceps are used to pull the vas up through the incision or puncture. To sever the vas deferens, the surgeon may:
- cut and tie, removing a short portion of tissue
- use clips
- use electrocautery to seal the ends of the vas deferens.

All of these techniques seem to produce equally good results.

Sperm will still be produced by the testicles and may build up behind the closed end of the vas. The accumulation can sometimes

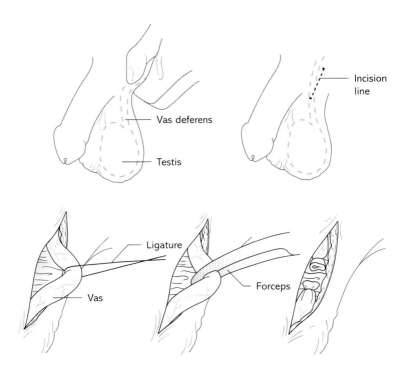

Figure 9.1 The standard vasectomy technique.

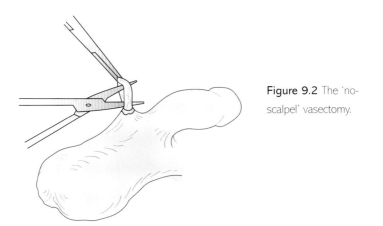

Figure 9.2 The 'no-scalpel' vasectomy.

be painful. Fortunately, sperm have a short lifespan; they soon die off and are absorbed by the body. Some surgeons may leave open one end of the vas deferens, closing only the section that connects with the penis. This allows sperm to spill and not accumulate in the delicate epididymis. Although a vasectomy that closes off only one end may be more easily reversible, it also has a somewhat greater chance of failure.

The 'no-scalpel' method, developed in China in the 1970s, is associated with a greatly reduced risk of hemorrhage. The approach takes only about 10 minutes and causes considerably less soreness, bleeding and bruising afterwards.

Most vasectomies take about 20 minutes. After a brief recovery period at the clinic, men are advised to rest at home for 24 hours to allow the incision to heal. Men who do physical labor are generally advised to wait for 1 week before going back to strenuous work. All men who have had vasectomies should wear an athletic support or jockey shorts for 4–6 weeks to support the scrotum until it is completely healed. The rule for having intercourse after a vasectomy is to wait until it feels comfortable, anywhere from a few days to 2 weeks.

Efficacy

Vasectomy is highly effective and should not be considered reversible. Although it is possible to repair the occluded vas, this requires delicate microsurgery, which is not always successful.

A typical first-year failure rate for vasectomy is 0.5–1.0%. Pregnancies can result from:

- unprotected intercourse before the reproductive tract has been totally emptied of the sperm present when the surgery was performed
- a closed vas reconnecting
- accidental interruption of a structure other than the vas deferens in the sterilization procedure, leaving the vas intact.

Reversibility

Like tubal occlusions for women, vasectomies can sometimes be reversed successfully. As the diameter of the inner canal of the vas deferens is approximately that of a pinpoint, a surgeon must use a microscope when rejoining the ends of these almost invisible tubes.

Because this requires major surgery, it is done under general anesthesia, is expensive and requires a long recovery time. Patency of the tube may be established, but pregnancy may still not occur because of the development of antisperm antibodies. Pregnancy rates following a reversal procedure vary from 16 to 79%, with the majority of clinics achieving a success rate close to 50%.

Because successful reversal is difficult, the decision to opt for male sterilization should be given long, careful thought and be accompanied by good counseling. Before undergoing this operation, it is essential for a man to feel comfortable with the fact that a vasectomy is permanent. Spousal consent is not required, but it is a good idea for a man to include his partner in the decision-making process, if possible.

Contraindications

In the WHO *Medical Eligibility Criteria*, male surgical sterilization warrants only just over one page. If there is local skin infection, systemic infection or gastroenteritis, filariasis or an intrascrotal mass, the WHO tables recommend delaying the vasectomy until the problem has resolved or been investigated. Caution is recommended in the presence of a large varicocele or hydrocele, cryptorchidism or previous scrotal injury (any of which may make surgery technically more difficult), or if the man is diabetic (since wound healing may be compromised). Vasectomy should be undertaken in an appropriately specialized unit if the man has AIDS or a coagulation disorder, or requires a simultaneous hernia repair.

Complications

Complications after vasectomy occur in only a fraction of procedures. They include:

- hematoma (1.6%)
- infection (1.5–3.4%)
- epididymitis (1.4%)
- sperm granulomas (0.3%).

Sperm granulomas (nodules caused by the presence of sperm that have leaked from one end of the severed vas) need treatment only if

---

Key points – male sterilization and hormonal methods for men

- Vasectomy is highly effective, and the procedure is simple.
- A variety of techniques for interrupting the vas deferens exist; they appear to be equally effective.
- 'No-scalpel' vasectomy is associated with less bleeding and pain than other methods.
- No good evidence substantiates the suggested association between vasectomy and prostate and testicular cancer.
- Although fertility can be restored after vasectomy, success rates are low.
- Hormonal methods of contraception for men based on a combination of testosterone and a progestogen are likely to become available in the next 10 years.

---

they are painful. This may involve removing the vas deferens so that sperm do not reach the granuloma.

Side effects

Although an association between vasectomy and prostate and testicular cancer has been suggested, there is no good evidence to substantiate this and no biologically plausible reason for an association.

Future prospects

Vasectomy. Work has progressed in China to develop reversible vasectomy using removable silicone plugs inserted into the vas deferens.

Hormonal methods. For a number of years, efforts have concentrated on developing hormonal methods for men, and the prospects for a method becoming available within the next 10 years seem good. Progestogens, antiandrogens and GnRH antagonists will all inhibit spermatogenesis, but also interfere with sexual function, requiring the addition of testosterone to maintain libido and erectile function. There is, as yet, no orally active testosterone formulation that can be used for this approach, so implants or injections must be used. Side effects of testosterone regimens include changes in serum lipids, with a theoretical increase in the risk of cardiovascular disease, and also possible prostate hypertrophy and cancer. Now the shortcomings of this approach have been recognized, efforts have turned to developing drugs that interfere with the maturation rather than with the production of sperm, thus avoiding interference with endogenous secretion of testosterone and its physiological functions.

Key references

Anderson RA, Baird DT. Male contraception. *Endocr Rev* 2002; 23:735–62.

Cook LA, Vliet H, Pun A, Gallo MF. Vasectomy occlusion techniques for male sterilization. *Cochrane Database Syst Rev* 2004;3: CD003991. *The Cochrane Library*, issue 4. Chichester: John Wiley & Sons, 2004 (www.thecochranelibrary.com).

Jamieson DJ, Costello C, Trussell J et al. The risk of pregnancy after vasectomy. *Obstet Gynecol* 2004; 103:848–50.

McDonald SW. Is vasectomy harmful to health? *Br J Gen Pract* 1997;47: 381–6.

Nieschlag E, Zitzmann M, Kamischke A. Use of progestins in male contraception. *Steroids* 2003;68:965–72.

Peterson HB, Howards SS. Vasectomy and prostate cancer: the evidence to date. *Fertil Steril* 1998; 70:201–3.

Pollack AE. Long-term consequences of female and male sterilization. *Contemp Obstet Gynecol* 1993; August:45–6.

Royal College of Obstetricians and Gynaecologists (RCOG). *Male and female sterilisation. Evidence-Based Clinical Guidelines* No. 4. 2nd edn. London: RCOG, 2004.

Schulman LM, Coulson AH, Mandel JS et al. Health status of American men – a study of post-vasectomy sequelae: results. *J Clin Epidemiol* 1993;46:697–958.

Turner L, Conway AJ, Jimenez M et al. Contraceptive efficacy of a depot progestin and androgen combination in men. *J Clin Endocrinol Metab* 2003;88:4659–67.

Useful resources

World Health Organization (WHO)
Reproductive Health Resources
www.who.int/reproductive-
health/publications/index.htm
WHO *Medical Eligibility Criteria
for Contraceptive Use*, 3rd edn,
2004
www.who.int/reproductive-health/
publications/MEC_3/mec.pdf
WHO *Selected Practice
Recommendations for
Contraceptive Use*, 2nd edn, 2004
www.who.int/reproductive-health/
publications/rhr_02_7/spr.pdf

US Food and Drug Administration
www.fda.gov

Faculty of Family Planning and
Reproductive Healthcare
Royal College of Obstetricians and
Gynaecologists, London, UK
www.ffprhc.org.uk
(website includes a number of
helpful, evidence-based guidance
documents)

Contraception Online
Baylor College of Medicine,
Houston, Texas, USA
(a resource for clinicians,
researchers and educators)
www.contraceptiononline.org

The Alan Guttmacher Institute
(a non-profit organization for
sexual and reproductive health)
www.agi-usa.org

Geneva Foundation for Medical
Education and Research
(lists of useful resources)
www.gfmer.ch/Guidelines/
Family_planning/Family_planning_
contraception.htm *and*
www.gfmer.ch/Guidelines/
Family_planning/Family_planning_
mt.htm

Association of Reproductive Health
Professionals
www.arhp.org
www.arhp.org/contraception
resources
www.arhp.org/choosing

Index

Your opinion matters – and that's a(nother) fact!

We hope that this *Fast Facts* book is just what you were looking for.

Our goal is to provide you with the ultimate medical handbook series – a series that blends quality of authorship and content with clear, concise design to serve you better than any other book in both study and practice.

Just as best practice evolves through the application of evidence, we want *Fast Facts* to evolve to meet the changing needs of the multidisciplinary healthcare team and those they care for.

And so your opinion really does matter!

If you have recommendations to make that will help us better meet your needs then we want to hear them, however left-field they are.

We are waiting for your message at:

feedback@fastfacts.com

Fast Facts:
- more than 60 titles and 40 on the way to cover all of medicine
- 1.4 million copies sold
- translated into 8 languages
- widely reviewed in the world's leading medical journals
- authors from 12 different nations, with at least 2 nationalities on each book

www.fastfacts.com

What the reviewers say:

This book is a little goldmine and is very good value for money

On *Fast Facts – Endometriosis, 2nd edn,* in *Medical Journal of Australia* 2004

concise and well written and accompanied by numerous excellent color illustrations... an excellent little book! Score: 100 - 5 Stars

On *Fast Facts – Sexual Dysfunc*
in *Doody's Health Sciences Review,* 2

this small volume is pleasingly pithy, erudite and accessible, as well as being helpfully informative

On *Fast Facts – Bipolar Disorder, 2nd edn,* in *Medical Journal of Australia* 2004

a timely and accessible book...
a worthwhile and handy tool for medical students

On *Fast Facts – Dyspepsia,* in *Digestive and Liver Disease* 36, 2004

provides a lot of information in a concise and easily accessible format...
a practical guide to managing most lower respiratory tract infections

On *Fast Facts – Respiratory Tract Infection,*
in *Respiratory Care* 49(1), 2004

an invaluable guide to the latest thinking

On *Fast Facts – Irritable Bowel Syndrome,* in *Update,* 4 September 2003

a rapid guide to understanding dementia...
value for money and I would definitely recommend it

On *Fast Facts – Dementia,* in *South African Medical Journal* 93(10), 2003

xcellent coverage of symptoms nd diagnosis

On *Fast Facts – Dyspepsia*, in *Update*, 19 June, 2003

will likely be read cover to cover in just one or two sittings by all who are fortunate enough to obtain a copy

On *Fast Facts – Benign Prostatic Hyperplasia*, 4th edn, in *Doody's Health Sciences Review*, Dec 2002

explains the important facts and demonstrates the levels of "good practice" that can be achieved

On *Fast Facts – Minor Surgery*, in *Journal of the Royal Society for the Promotion of Health* 122(3), 2002

a splendid publication

On *Fast Facts – Sexually Transmitted Infections*, in *Journal of Antimicrobial Chemotherapy* 49, 2002

I would highly recommend it without reservation... 5 stars!

On *Fast Facts – Psychiatry Highlights 2001–02*, in *Doody's Health Sciences Review*, Sept 2002

I enthusiastically recommend this stimulating, short book which should be required reading for all clinicians

On *Fast Facts – Irritable Bowel Syndrome*, in *Gastroenterology* 120(6), 2001

***** outstanding

On *Fast Facts – HIV in Obstetrics and Gynecology*, in *Journal of Pelvic Surgery*, 2001

www.fastfacts.com

FAST FACTS

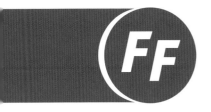

An outstandingly successful independent medical handbook series

Over one million copies sold

- Written by world experts
- Concise and practical
- Up-to-date
- Designed for ease of reading and reference
- Copiously illustrated with useful photographs, diagrams and charts

Our aim for *Fast Facts* is to be **the world's most respected medical handbook series**. Feedback on how to make titles even more useful is always welcome (feedback@fastfacts.com).

Fast Facts titles include

Acne	Headaches (second edition)
Allergic Rhinitis	Hyperlipidemia (third edition)
Asthma (second edition)	Hypertension (second edition)
Benign Gynecological Disease (second edition)	Inflammatory Bowel Disease
Benign Prostatic Hyperplasia (fourth edition)	Irritable Bowel Syndrome (second edition)
Bipolar Disorder	Menopause (second edition)
Bladder Cancer (second edition)	Minor Surgery
Bleeding Disorders	Multiple Sclerosis
Brain Tumors	Osteoporosis (third edition)
Breast Cancer (third edition)	Parkinson's Disease
Celiac Disease	Prostate Specific Antigen (second edition)
Chronic Obstructive Pulmonary Disease	Psoriasis
Colorectal Cancer (second edition)	Respiratory Tract Infection (second edition)
Contraception (second edition)	Rheumatoid Arthritis
Dementia	Schizophrenia (second edition)
Depression	Sexual Dysfunction
Disorders of the Hair and Scalp	Sexually Transmitted Infections
Dyspepsia (second edition)	Smoking Cessation
Eczema and Contact Dermatitis	Soft Tissue Rheumatology
Endometriosis (second edition)	Superficial Fungal Infections
Epilepsy (second edition)	Travel Medicine
Erectile Dysfunction (third edition)	Urinary Continence (second edition)
Gynecological Oncology	Urinary Stones

Orders

To order via the website, or to find regional distributors, please go to
www.fastfacts.com

For telephone orders, please call +44 (0)1752 202301 (Europe) or
800 538 1287 (North America, toll free)